Basic Laboratory Methods for Pharmacology and Toxicology

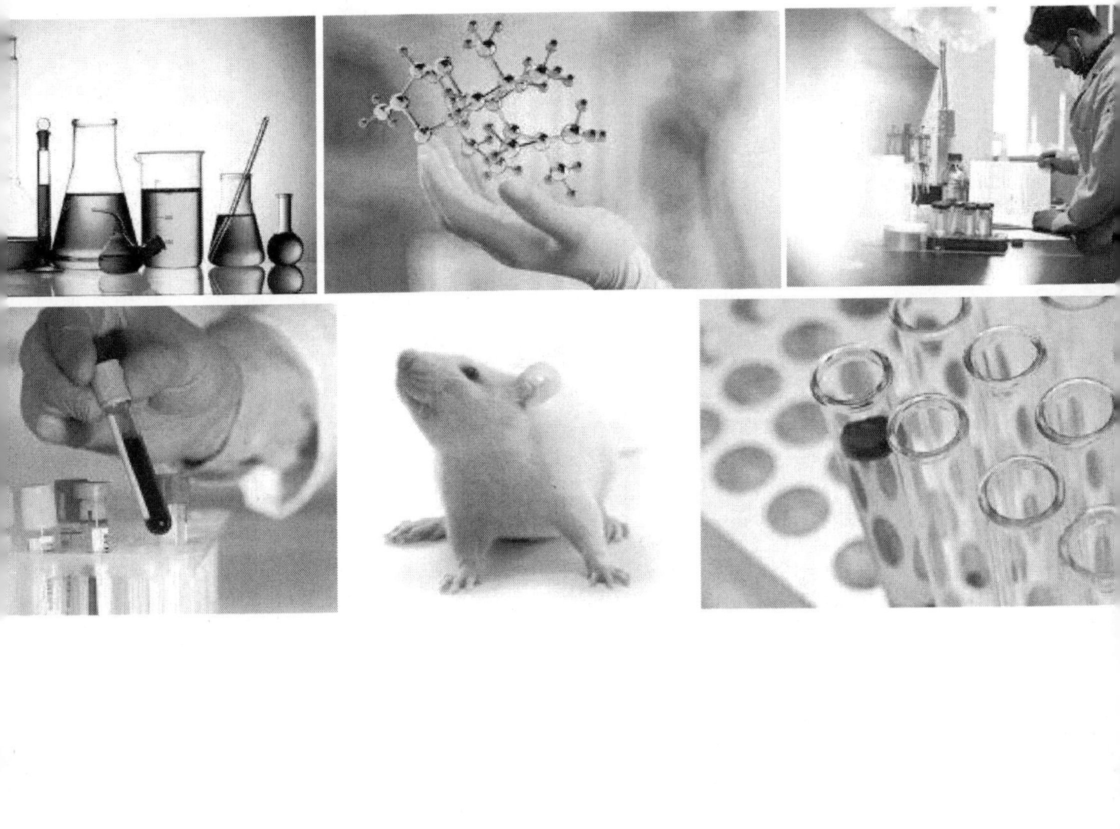

The Editors

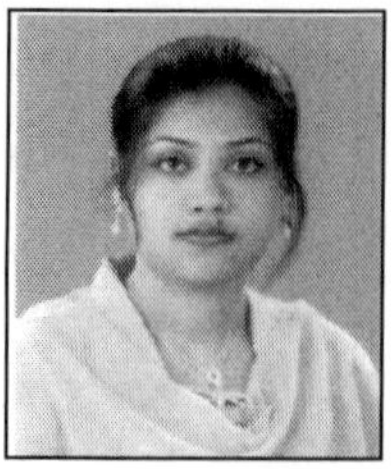

Sabrina Sharmin is currently Assistant Professor in Department of Pharmacy, Brac University, Bangladesh. She received her Ph. D (Biophysics) in 2018 from Shizuoka University under the scope of MEXT scholarship, MS degree (Pharmaceutical Chemistry) in 2008 and Bachelor degree in Pharmacy from University of Dhaka, Bangladesh. She had done her postdoctoral training from 2018 to 2019 in Shizuoka University, Japan. In 2020, she had joined as a Postdoc Associate in Pharmacology department, University of Minnesota, United States America. She acquired a Travel Award in 61st Annual Meeting of Biophysical Society, New Orleans, Louisiana, USA. From 2008 to 2014, she worked in multinational pharmaceutical company Sanofi Bangladesh Ltd as a quality control specialist. During her doctoral and postdoctoral study, she had investigated interactions of peptides/ proteins with bio membranes as well as *E. coli* cells and tried to develop new imaging methods to investigate structures, functions, and dynamics of bio membranes and cells, and reveal elementary processes of the dynamics of these biomolecular super-assemblies to elucidate mechanisms of their functions. In nano biotechnology laboratory, She worked on developing fluorescence based nano composite for the detection of viruses which I published in 2020.

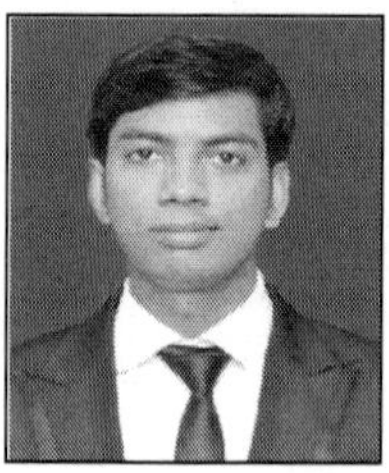

Manish Kumar Verma is currently pursuing Ph. D in Veterinary Pharmacology and Toxicology from the College of Veterinary and Animal Sciences, G. B. Pant University of Agriculture and Technology, Pantnagar, Uttarakhand. He completedB.V.Sc and A.H (2016) and M.V.Sc (2018) in Veterinary Pharmacology and Toxicology also from the same Institute. He joined as Junior Research Fellow in the project entitled "Monitoring of Drug Residues and Environmental Pollutants" by the Indian Council for Agricultural Research (ICAR), New Delhi. He served as a Guest faculty (2018 to 2019) in the department of Veterinary Pharmacology and Toxicology, College of Veterinary Science and Animal Husbandry, N.D. University of Agriculture and Technology. Kumarganj, Ayodhya, Uttar Pradesh. He has over the years investigated the immunomodulatory and antioxidant property of phytochemicals and Nano vaccine of Salmonella. He is currently working on the evaluation of effects of fipronil on xenobiotic metabolism.

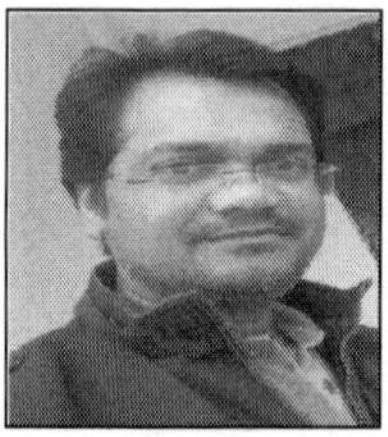

Dr. R.P. Diwakar is currently working as Assistant Professor in Department of Veterinary Microbiology, College of Veterinary Science and A.H, Acharya Narendra Deva University of Agriculture and Technology, Kumarganj, Ayodhya (Utter-Pradesh) He obtained, Undergraduate degree from the GBPUA and T, Pantnagar (U.K) in the year 2004 and master's degree in Veterinary Microbiology from the College of Veterinary Science and Animal Husbandry, NDUA and T, Kumarganj, Faizabad in year 2006. Dr. Diwakar was join as SRF in research unit, Institute of Biotechnology, Patwadagar district Nainital (U.K) in year 2006 and in year 2007 join in teaching as a teaching Associate in Department of Veterinary Microbiology in NDUA and T, Kumarganj and in Oct. 2007 join the state government job Veterinary officer. In year 2012,join as a Assistant professor in Department of Veterinary Microbiology, His research interests is mainly Enterobacteria associated with calf diarrhoea specially E.coli. Prepared total 07 manuals for students in different courses of Veterinary Microbiology and published more than 38 Research articles/16 Review articles/02 Short communication, lead papers 09, 16 Popular articles and case study 06. Written 05 book in Veterinary Microbiology courses for B.V.Sc and A.H, MVSc, students and 02 books for animal owners and para vets, gotseveral awards from the different scientific societies of national and international forum and also work as Editorial members/Reviewer in different National and International journal.

Basic Laboratory Methods for Pharmacology and Toxicology

— *Chief Editor* —

Sabrina Sharmin

MS, Ph.D, PDF
Assistant Professor
Department of Pharmacy, Brac University, Bangladesh

— *Editors* —

Manish Kumar Verma

M.V.Sc
Research Scholar
Department of Veterinary Pharmacology and Toxicology
G.B. Pant University of Agriculture and Technology,
Pantnagar, Uttarakhand, India

R.P. Diwakar

M.V.Sc
Assistant Professor
Department of Veterinary Microbiology
Acharya Narendra Deva University of Agriculture Technology,
Kumarganj, Ayodhya, Uttar Pradesh, India

BIOTECH

2022

BIOTECH BOOKS®

ISBN 978-81-7622-495-6

Published by: **BIOTECH BOOKS®**
4762-63/23, Ansari Road, Darya Ganj,
New Delhi - 110 002
Phone: 09899295259, 011-43003222
E-mail: biotechbooks@yahoo.co.in
Website: www.biotechbooks.in

Typeset at: **Classic Computer Services**
Delhi - 110 035

Printed at: **Replika Press Pvt. Ltd.**

PRINTED IN INDIA

ILRI
INTERNATIONAL LIVESTOCK RESEARCH INSTITUTE

CGIAR

1st Floor, C-Block, NASC Complex,
New Delhi 110012, India
Mobile: +91-9483527849
Tel: +91 11 25847885, 25609800,
Email r.habibar@cgiar.org

15 February 2021

Foreword

I am pleased to go through the content of the First Edition of the book entitled "Basic Laboratory Methods for Pharmacology and Toxicology" edited by Dr. Sabrina Sharmin and Dr. Manish Kumar Verma and their team. I find that the work would be extremely useful for new budding undergraduate (UG) and post-graduate (PG) students. This book covers the basic laboratory methods, which are important for the B.V.Sc. & A.H. students (All-in-One) and also for entrance examination like JRF, SRF, ASRB, CSIR (NET) and other competitive examinations. The current era needs skilled researchers with amicable skillset for augmenting and sustaining growth of science, which is only possible through quality education.

I am sure that students and researchers, not only medical sciences but other allied science students will also be benefited.

My cordial blessings to the editor and co-editors for their comprehensive publication!

(Dr. H. Rahman)
Regional Representative for South Asia,
International Livestock Research Institute &
Former Deputy Director General (Animal Sciences),
Indian Council of Agricultural Research (ICAR), New Delhi &
Former Director, ICAR – National Institute of Veterinary Epidemiology
and Disease Informatics (NIVEDI), Bengaluru

Preface

Knowledge of Pharmacology and Toxicology continue to move ahead on many fronts. In recent years the laboratory methodology of pharmacology and toxicology has undergone a sea of changes with the development of new techniques of preparation and testing the samples. The major objective of this book is to provide students and researchers, collective information about basic laboratory methodology of pharmacology and toxicology in a simple and lucid language and thus the guiding tools for them. Students and researchers who have completed their basic courses based on this book should be able to approach directly, with a sound knowledge of basic laboratory techniques.

In the book most portions deal with the research laboratory procedure of kinetics of drug design and elementary pharmacological test. It contains methods of handling, drug administration and collection of blood from laboratory animals, methods for detection of antimicrobial resistanceand minimum concentration of antibiotics, pharmacokinetic study design, tissue organ bath system, general diagnostic toxicology, reproductive and developmental toxicity assessment, genotoxicity assessment, immunoassays, and computeraided drug design and methods of euthanasia. Within each chapter, emphasis is placed on discussion of drug development procedures. Different types of methodology of pharmacology as well as toxicology have added to enrich this book.

This book is a first attempt by the authors. We have tried our best to make it flawless. This book will be much useful as a source of quick reference for students and researchers. However, we would appreciate suggestions and comments from our valued readers to make it more informative and useful in the future edition.

Sabrina Sharmin

Manish Kumar Verma

R.P. Diwakar

Contents

List of Contributors

Methods of Laboratory Animal Handling and Drug Administration	Methods of Collection of Blood From Laboratory Animals
Mehrukh Zehravi, *M.Pharm, RPh* *Lecturer, Department of Clinical Pharmacy, Prince Sattam Bin Abdul Aziz University, Alkharj-Riyadh, Saudi Arabia*	***Dr. Satuti Sharma,*** *M.V.Sc* *Ph.D. Scholar, Department of Veterinary Pathology, Sher-e-Kashmir University of Agricultural Sciences and Technology, Jammu, India*
Methods for Detection of Antimicrobial Resistance	**Determination of the Minimum Inhibitory Concentration of Antibiotics**
Garima Pandey, *Ph.D* *Department of Veterinary Microbiology, G.B. Pant University of Agriculture and Technology, Pantnagar, Uttarakhand, India*	***R.P. Diwakar,*** *M.V.Sc* *Assistant Professor, Department of Veterinary Microbiology C.V.Sc. and A.H., ANDUAT, Kumarganj, Ayodhya, Uttar Pradesh, India*
Pharmacokinetic Study Design	**Tissue Organ Bath System**
Dr. Neelam Dinodia, *M.V.Sc* *Ph.D. Scholar, Department of Veterinary Pharmacology and Toxicology NDVSU, Jabalpur, Madhya Pradesh, India*	***Rishikant,*** *M.V.Sc* *Assistant Professor, Department of Veterinary Pharmacology and Toxicology, C.V.Sc. and A.H., ANDUAT, Kumarganj, Ayodhya, Uttar Pradesh, India*

General Diagnostic Toxicology ***Anand Kumar,*** *Ph.D.* *Department of Veterinary Medicine, G.B. Pant University of Agriculture and Technology, Pantnagar, Uttarakhand, India*	**Reproductive and Developmental Toxicity Assessment** ***Abhishek Pandey,*** *M.V.Sc.* *Ph.D. Scholar, Department of Veterinary Pharmacology and Toxicology, G.B. Pant University of Agriculture and Technology, Pantnagar, Uttarakhand, India*
Genotoxicity Assessment ***Dr. Aman Kamboj,*** *Ph.D* *Assistant Professor, Department of Veterinary Physiology and Biochemistry, G.B. Pant University of Agriculture and Technology, Pantnagar, India*	**Immunoassays** ***Aakansha Tiwari,*** *Ph.D* *Department of Veterinary Microbiology, G.B. Pant University of Agriculture and Technology, Pantnagar, Uttarakhand, India*
Computer Aided Drug Design ***Maymoonah Binte Amanullah,*** *M. Pharm.* *Research Scholar, Department of Pharmacy, Primeasia University, Dhaka, Bangladesh*	**Methods of Euthanasia** ***Swati Rawat,*** *Ph.D.* *Assistant Professor, MIT, Moradabad, Uttar Pradesh, India*

Chapter 1

Methods of Laboratory Animal Handling and Drug Administration

Around 50–100 million vertebrate animals are used in experiments annually for the study of chemical, pharmaceuticals, medical, biological, toxicology and genetics. The course of administration depends greatly on the property and the intent of the test material. Each administration should be carried out with an understanding of the substance's chemical and physical attributes. Demerits and merits are associated with all routes, including absorption, bioavailability and drug metabolism. Their pH, viscosity, concentration, sterility, pyrogenicity, toxicity and existence of toxic substances should be considered seriously. The scientist/investigator will be equipped with knowledge of possible administration methods and different techniques, and also awareness of deposition and fate of the administered drug. Thus the route has to be selected before any research project begins.

Proper restraint, which lessens stress and tends to increase successful treatment, is perhaps the most relevant technique when treating mice. Personnel handling laboratory animals should be adequately trained in monitoring and preservation, are able to achieve compliance for safe use and meet a technically high standard for experimental animals. More practice can yield functional and accurate results. Laboratory animals should be protected from pain, misery, discomfort or enduring long-term damage during administration, or at least pain and discomfort must be minimized. There is a significant discouragement for some of the injections (such as footpad injection) and case by case, when appropriate, justified.[1]

Characteristics and Attributes of Administration

Handling and Restraining of the Animal – Procedures with Care

The most critical method for appropriate administration is effective handling and retention. Adequate constraints contribute to efficient administration and vary in routes. There are two types of manual restraints, one using both hands and the other held by one hand. Required gloves must be chosen to wear since manual retention is used for injecting generally.[2]

a) Manual Restraint (Double Handed)

In manual restraint, while using mice its been lifted and being placed on the flat surface or lid of the cage can be used instead with the base of the tail by using one handedly by pulling back its tail gently and softly. Moreover, by using the index finger and thumb of the other hand its then picked firmly by using the scruff of the neck behind the ears. Its then from the first hand, the tail is transferred and fixed to the other hand between the palm and the ring finger for restraining.

b) Single Handed Restraint

The mouse is positioned on the firm surface by the thumb and front finger of the preferred hand. The palm and the middle finger, the finger and/or little finger instantly grasp the tail and remove the thumb and forefinger. However, the thumb and forefinger, the skin fold from the scruff of the back is immediately gripped. The tail is supported by the palm and forefinger in order to prevent the movement of the hind legs, while the left hind leg is firmly held between the ring and baby finger in that way mouse is being restrained by the left hand.

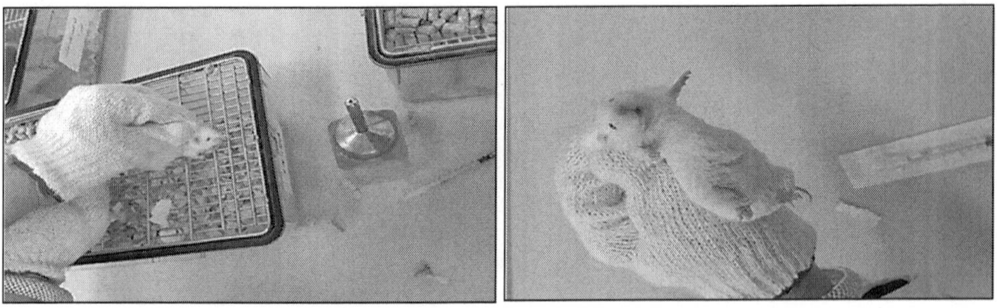

Figure 1.1: Shows Procedure for Manual Restraint.

Administration Site

The most popular routes are subcutaneous, intraperitoneal or intravenous injections, among several possible ways of administration of substances to the mouse. It is not advised to use the intramuscular method as the muscles seems too small. Several locations, such as Freund's full adjuvant footpad injection, the intraspenic and intra-lymph node injector sites, are actually inappropriate.[1]

Site Preparation

If required before cleansing the skin with alcohol or disinfectant, the region of administration shall be either clipped or washed with warm water. When aseptic skin is desired, a 3-stage surgical treatment must be performed, preceded after the fur clipping: soap process, alcoholic rinsing and surgical preparation. Until operation, the skin is dried instantly.[1] In certain situations, the first use of a local anesthetic would be to deal with pain.

Preparation, Solubility and Safety of Solutions

Especially in the context of Parenteral Injections, the test substances, solutions and equipment must be prepared aseptically and should be pyrogens free. Once administered, live organisms or cells should be free of contamination. To avoid tissue damage and to give an accurate dosage, the toxicity, volume and method of administration of the substance should be taken into account. In the majority of cases, the following solvents or equipment is considered to be acceptable and do not significantly affect drug activity attributing to their own intrinsic properties *i.e.* water, 0.85 per cent sodium chloride with water, not over 10 per cent Tween 80 with water, 0.25 per cent methylcellulose or carboxymethylcellulose with water, 50 per cent polyethylene glycol with water and corn oil; vegetable oil; peanut oil (oral and i/m route only). By keeping the administered volume small, the lowest percentage of lower alcohols, glycols, phosphate buffered saline (PBS) and acetones can be used. Absorption is expected to be delayed for lipid-soluble substances as they can only be dissolved in oil. Intravenously oil soluble drugs *i.e.*, 15 per cent oil-water emulsions with the help of lecithin as emulsifiers were effectively and successfully given.[3]

While distilled water may be administered within certain circumstances, saline is preferred since water for injection injected by subcutaneously route causes pain and by intravenous route causes hemolysis. For intravenous injection of suspended material, the separation of the particle can be done by using the process of filtration to avoid embolism.[3] The fluid temperature must be elevated at minimum to room or more even before application, since it is uncomfortable to administer the cold fluid.

Injected Solution's pH and Concentration of Substances

Most of the administered solutions pH ranges up to 4.5 to 8.0. High pH can be accepted for oral administration, but alkaline solutions are not very well handled. Owing to the buffering effect of blood and blood flow dilution following intra-muscular and then sub-cutaneous routes, a somewhat huge pH range is indicated for intravenous administration. Whenever low or high pH solutions are injected intravenously, the injection rate is regulated gradually and carefully taking steps to keep substances from going outside the vein.[3]

Without significantly affecting the final outcome, the concentration may differ in a relatively broad range. It is obviously preferable at lower concentrations.[4]

Volume and Frequency of Administration

The volume of the injection is restricted by both the substance's toxicity and mouse size. This should be kept to a minimum. The animal can suddenly be shocked by excessive quantities of solution. In order to eliminate undue stress, the rate of administration should be restricted. Hemodynamic shifts and pulmonary edema can happen when solutions are given intravenously, whereas extremely rapid injections can contribute to heart failure and lethality.[5]

Guidelines for Maximal Administration Volumes (in milliliters) and Needle Size

Oral	*Subcutaneous*	*Intraperitoneal*	*Intravenous*	*Intradermal*	*Intramuscular*	*Intracerebral*	*Intranasal*
0.2	2–3 (scruff) 0.2 (inguinal)	2-3	0.2	0.05	0.05	<0.03	<0.02
<22G		**<23G**	**<25G**	**<26G**	**25-27G**	**<27G**	

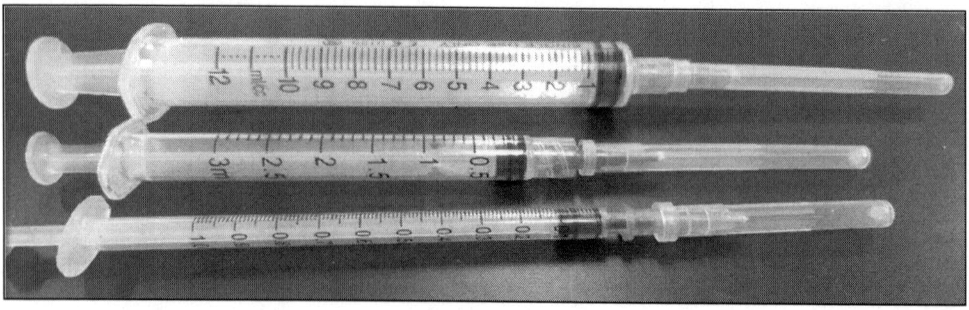

Figure 1.2: Shows different Types of Syringes *i.e.* 10ml, 3ml and 1ml

Route of Administration

The use of substances in laboratory animals is often a critical component of experimental design. Infectious agents, specific therapeutics including vaccines, antimicrobials, pharmacological agents, anesthetics, analgesics, chemical evaluation, radiocontrast agents, electrolytes and other fluids used for the administered substances.

The route they take, administration of frequency and volume, duration of treatment, pH, safety, homogeneity and osmolality of the administered substance, use of vehicles or solvents for the delivery of substances that cannot be delivered in a solid state, how solution is being prepared, considering parenteral administration of the drug specifically involves sterility, dosing devices and animal containment needed for particular distribution routes. Therefore, researchers should be aware of possible adverse effects associated with the administration of substances to clear up any confusion with other aspects of the design of studies and to ensure a proper interpretation of the research results.

There are wide varieties of routes employed by which substances are administered to laboratory animals. The key factor determining the route chosen is whether the agent is administered for a local or systemic (enteral or parenteral) effect.

- Enteral route (digestive): oral (to the mouth) or gavage (esophageal, gastric, or nasogastric)
- Parenteral route: intravenous, epicutaneous, intradermal.

The selection of a given route depending on the objective of the study may affect regulatory requirements, for *e.g.*: in nonclinical safety testing, the route of delivery for the animal should be close to the intended route of human administration.[6]

1. Entral Route of Administration

In laboratory animal testing and research it is normal to directly administer substances in the mouth, blended into diets or other nutritional products by orogastric gavage. Enema or suppositories are less common in animals as per rectum delivering substances than in humans. The benefits of enteral administration are that large quantities of non-sterile substances or solution can be provided and that this route can administer the pH as low as 3. On the other side, this path has very little toleration of alkaline solutions. It is necessary to realize when using the oral route that the materials may be annihilated by gastric juices and that the food in the stomach affects both the order and the rate of gastric emptying. The absorption rate is significantly affected by their time in the stomach and it is directly related to the rate of transfer of substances from the stomach to the intestine. The methods commonly used for enteral administration is combining or mixing the substance or compound with drinking water and food or directly administering it with the help of gavage. Rectal administration can also be employed.[7]

a. Administration via Oral Route

The oral pathway is inexpensive, easy, and generally safe. Based on whether the drug is delivered, certain individuals may be conditioned for voluntary cooperation. Even though it is ideal to willingly consume the substance being administered, this dosing strategy may not always be effective in all animals or dosage groups or for long-term research due to individual preferences for flavors, palatability concerns, and behavioral changes over time. Oral dosage imitates the most commonly employed method of administering substances to humans evaluated for safety. Therefore administering substances in food and drinking water appears to be the easiest and simple method known in animals.

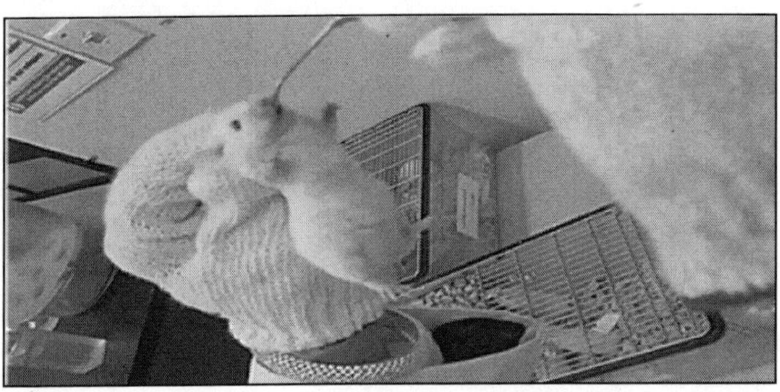

Figure 1.3: Oral Route of Administration.

The average food and water consumption of mouse should be identified before the procedure to measure the amount of material to be combined. Drugs when inserted orally, it is essential to ensure that test material-containing tablets or gelatin capsules are put well back in the mouth and the animal is swallowed to ensure a maximum dosage is obtained. To prevent regurgitation, the number and size of capsules or tablets issued should be proportional to the size of the animal being dosed.

b. Intra-Gastric via Gavage

Esophageal or gastric gavage is often used in experimental settings to facilitate reliable and correct treatment in specimens, rather than just incorporating substances through water or food.

Appropriate tubing measurements have always been chosen for orogastric or nasogastric gavage to minimize pain and to enhance substance distribution. For the enteral nutrition in rabbits and non-human primates, Naso-gastube is widely used for the administration of dose, usually consisting of 3 to 8 French pediatric feeding tubes. Tubes are usually measured and marked from external nares to the last rib.[8] A small quantity of xylocaine jelly can be placed directly at the end of the tubing to reduce pain before inserting the tubing 0.5 per cent of proparacaine HCl ophthalmic fluid is placed directly in the nares(Except when administered in the diet or in combination with food).[9]

Oral delivery of the substances usually requires a certain amount of restraint which is perhaps the most negative impact of a protocol in many animals, including rodents and non-human primates.[10] For oral administration, the smallest possible volume is advised to apply for optimal 5 mL/kg for all species (Table 1.1). If large volumes have to be delivered by gavage, animals that better withstand only a slower delivery rate. Researchers should then be trained and practiced prior to the initiation of a study to prevent adverse technical effects and to ensure that they are correctly, quickly and humanely conducted in laboratory animals. Oral gavage needs moderate technical expertise and confidence.

c. Rectal Administration

In laboratory animals, this approach is not widely utilized and substances can be delivered through a suppository or an enema. It's enteral to a GI tract but does not follow the oral route of delivery. A small gauge smooth, flexible tubing (3.5 French red rubber feeding tube) can be used for the preparation of drug solution for rectal administration. The tube used consists of smooth and curved margins while the end of the tubing is attached with the dosing syringe, ensuring that all air bubbles are eliminated. Restricting the volume of injection to 0.5 ml in the mouse and for rats the restriction leveled at 1-2 ml.[11]

2. Parentral Administration

Injection, infusion, topical application, and inhalation, as well as the implantation of osmotic pumping or controlled drug delivery pellets, encompasses the administration of substances other than the alimentary canal into the body. The solution comprises of large volumes are infused and small quantities are injected. The skin must be treated and penetrated by a needle in both cases. The most popular and major routes for administering drug substances or even suspensions into the mouse are subcutaneous, intraperitoneal and intravenous administration. The absorption rate relies on the proper selection of the route of delivery.

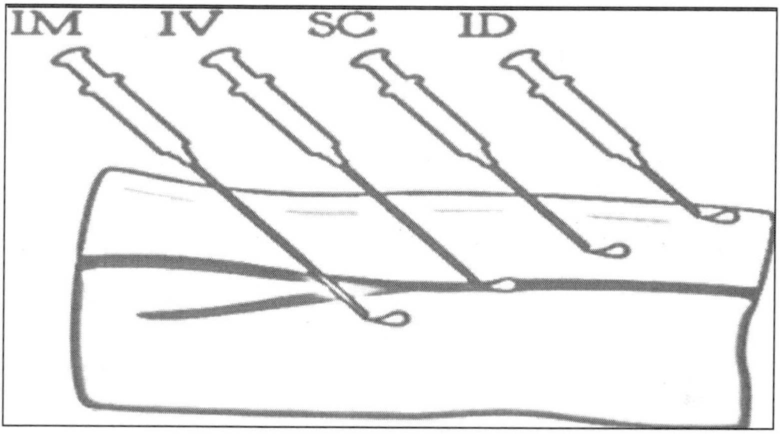

Figure 1.4: Different Routes of Skin Administration of Substances.

i. Administration via Intravenous Route

The most appropriate way to deliver drugs to animals is the intravenous route of delivery. Drugs are specifically supplied in blood vessels as a bolus or infusion through an acute or chronic basis. Precision electronic infusion pumps fitted with alarms to display flow discrepancies and Micro drop infusion sets are in use to assure the chronic intravenous administration of many substances.[12, 13] **Open in a separate window**

Before drug administration, prepares skin aseptically for percutaneous venous injection. Give the potential for major complications, such as visual impairment, cerebrovascular stroke, permanent motor deficits and limb gangrene. Purposeful intra-arterial administration of substances is to be prevented frequently and used strictly under particular experimental conditions.[14, 15] Intraosseous delivery of materials, notably crystalloid fluids, is used as an alternative to the intravenous route in hypovolemic patients with difficult to access or collapsed veins in human pediatric medicine and emergency avian and rabbit medicine.[16, 17]

Intraosseous administration procedure is complex and highly intrusive without the need for advanced training, with a substantial risk of post-process osteomyelitis, fatty embolization, iatrogenic dizziness and growth plate impairment and distress. Several oily agents such as cremaphorus and numerous alcohols, surfactants, and other vehicles as well as excipients can lead to intravenous hemolysis; these substances should be eliminated as much as possible or they must be first assessed *in vitro* for safety when intravenously introduced.[18, 19]

A proper vigilance of haemostasis is necessary to limit blood loss and the formation of a painful hematoma when the catheter or needle is withdrawn. In the event of drugs and infusions taken chronically, animals should be watched closely for signs like the overload of fluid or pulmonary oedema, particularly dyspnea and cyanosis.[20]

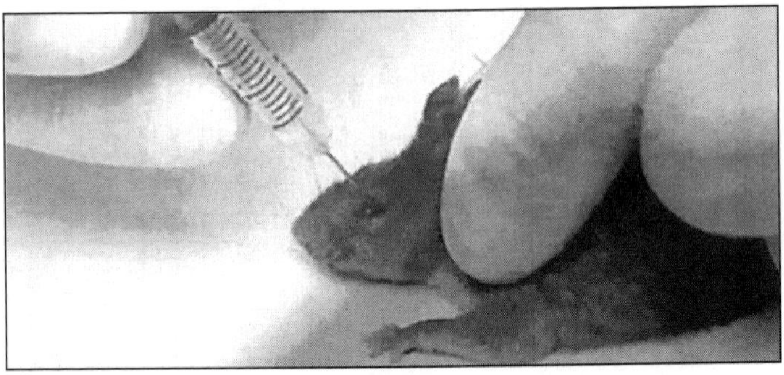

Figure 1.6: Intravenous Administration in to the Retro-orbital Sinus.

ii. Administration via Skin and Muscles

Those substances delivered epi-cutaneously can be applied directly over the skin surface for a specific topical effect. The degree to which substances are absorbed via the skin and enter into bloodstream circulation (*i.e.*, percutaneous or transdermal delivery) is based upon the region over which it is applied. The concentration of product material or vehicle lipid solubility intact surface of the skin, its thickness at the application site, the time it is in contact with the surface of the skin, and the degree of skins hydration and occlusion at the skin surface, therefore substances penetrate more quickly and rapidly in covered and well hydrated skin as compare to exposed or dry skin.[21]

Be vigilant to prevent the direct application of caustic or irritating material on skin and even certain substances that might cause local sensitivity reactions. The possibility for systemic toxicity should be considered in the topical administration of drugs, especially when the site is easy to access for grooming.[22] Applying thin layers of cream or ointment to the skin more frequently may be more effective for less systemic toxicity than applying thick layers less frequently. A similar route of administration is being represented by the transdermal or percutaneous delivery with the exception that products are used on the skin surface intentionally for absorption throughout the epithelial barrier all across the systemic circulation, typically by means of a patch. This process generally causes the substance to be delivered to very constant blood levels; percutaneous delivery is an appealing option to other routes in which frequent animal restraint unpleasant injections and extreme risks are prevented. Additionally, dosing requires to be stopped or in case adverse effects are observed, materials should readily be withdrawn from the skin surface. A skin for topical delivery is prepared. While using a transdermally delivery, the agent as well as system (for instance, patch) must be used in advance, where it is necessary to produce the desired effect, depending on the substance absorption pharmacokinetics. The product should be applied in such a manner so that it can be protected against ingestion and contamination and the toxicity signs should be known following accidental intakes by the animal.[23, 24]

Subcutaneously administered non-irritating substances can be administered as a quick affordable and simple method of administration of parenteral substances. Subcutaneously administered drugs, which have sustained effect, are often consumed at a lower rate than other parenteral routes.[55]

The administration of substances intramuscularly in large animals and humans is the typical parenteral method, perhaps avoided in reduced muscle mass in smaller species. The injections administered intravenously are probably the result of the rich vascular supply of consistent and quick absorption of substances. Intramuscularly smaller volumes are administered as compared to the amount delivered subcutaneously. Intramuscular administration of an irritant or an accidental injection of nerves could contribute to paralysis, necrosis of muscles, muscle sloughing and paresis. In the case of injections administered repeatedly inflammation and necrosis can be the resultant effect.[26]

iii. Administration via Epidural and Intrathecal Route

Substances can be delivered to the epidurally or within the subarachnoid (intrathecal) spaces of the spinal cord for rapid effects of substances on cerebrospinal tissues or meninges. The above technique prevents absorption problems that it does portrayed by the blood-brain barrier. Aseptic skin preparation that supersedes the site of the injection through the use of sterile needle insertion technology is essential. In comparison to intrathecal with epidural delivery the precise location of insertion of the needle and its injectate volumes will vary among species and multiple factors contribute to procedural success.[27] Epidural fat lipophilicity of the injected drug, intervertebral spaces injective leakage and extreme meningo-vertebral ligaments are all intended to limit or change the spreading of the content delivered by epidural or intrathecal pathways. After injecting the spinal needle, visualization of cerebro spinal fluid verifies that the needle is placed intrathecally. The administration of substances intrathecally or epidurally requires significant technical expertise and extensive knowledge regarding anesthesia, analgesia and anatomy of the vertebral column. Only well-trained personnel will perform these procedures.

Administration via Intraperitoneal Route

Substances are commonly injected into the peritoneal cavity in lab rodents but all seldom used in huge mammals and human beings. Intraperitoneal delivery is particularly used for the smallest animals that are complicated access intravenously and can be used to effectively deliver significant amounts of fluids. Intraperitoneally administered substance is typically delivered much slowly than intravenously delivered injection. Whereas intraperitoneal administration is regarded as a parenteral route of administration, the pharmacokinetics of the intraperitoneally delivered substances seem more like those seen following oral administration, because the main absorption route is through mesenteric vessels, draining in the portal veins and passing through the liver.[28]

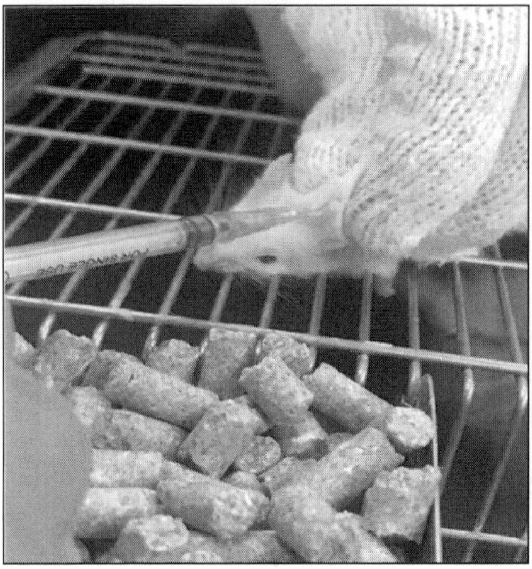

Figure 1.7: Subcutaneous Administration.

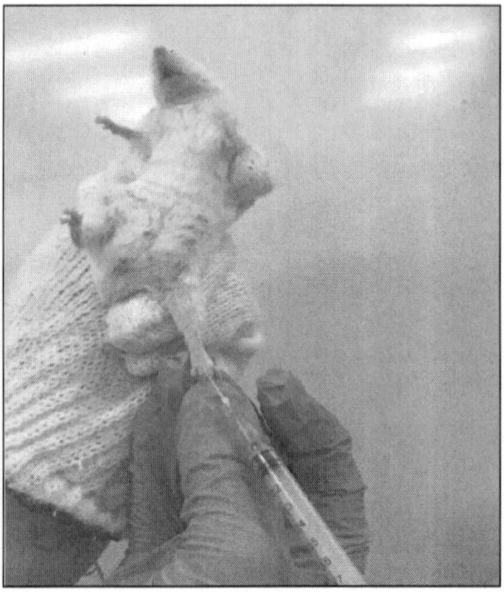

Figure 1.8: Intra Epidermal Administration.

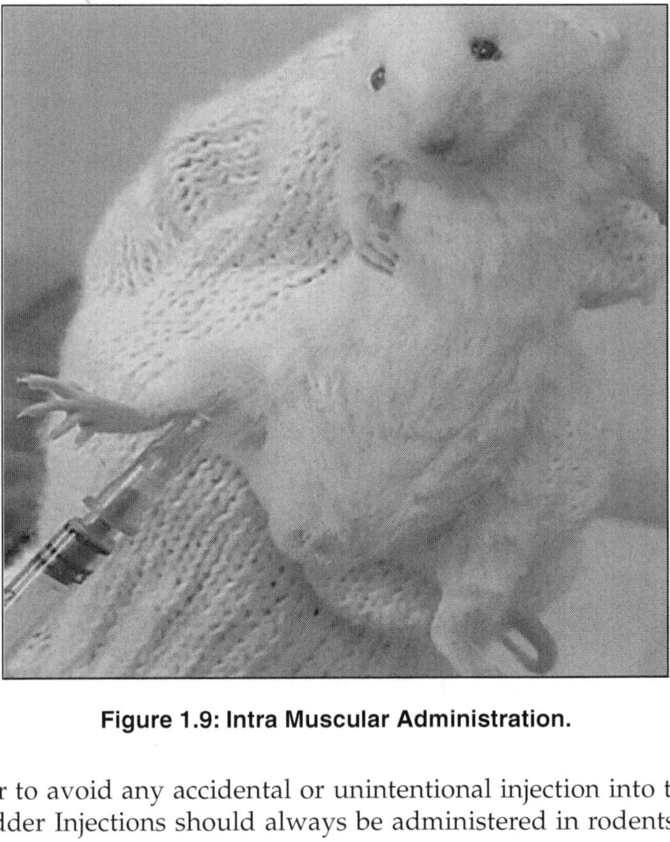

Figure 1.9: Intra Muscular Administration.

In order to avoid any accidental or unintentional injection into the caecum/ urinary bladder Injections should always be administered in rodents away from the midline, specifically in the lower right quadrant of the abdomen.[29] Prior to injecting make sure always to withdrawn the syringe plunger, in case of any fluid (*i.e.* urine, blood or digesta) spotted in the needle hub, it needs to be removed, replaced or repositioned before the injection. While injecting, puncturing the skin too deeply is the common mistake done usually which might result in subcutaneous administration rather than intraperitoneal delivery. Intraperitoneally injected irritating substances can cause painful ileus and peritonitis in rodents following adhesions.[30]

Peritoneal irritation may be avoided by injections of the same doses of chloral hydrate in less concentrated solutions.[31]

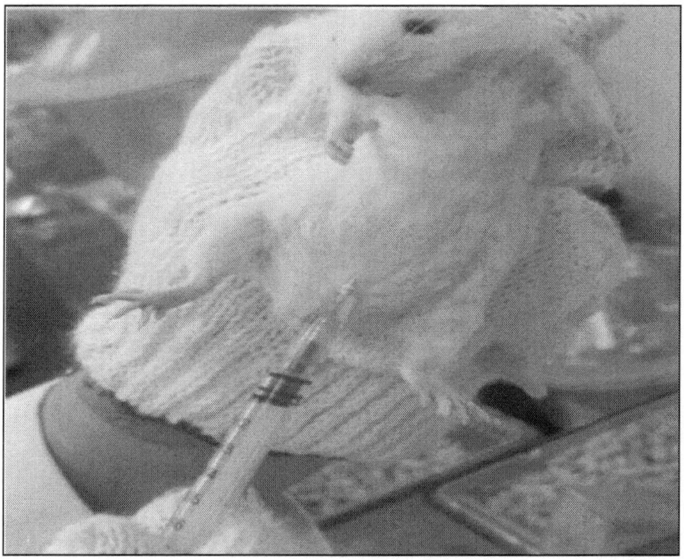

Figure 10: Intraperitoneal Administration.

iv. Administration via Intranasal Route

In research, animals are normally sedated or aestheticized in order to limit struggle and to sneez through the intranasal and intra-tracheal routes of delivery. The intranasally prescribed amounts in contrast to those on other routes are small in order to minimize suffocation and mortality risk. The procedure cannot be effective for symptoms of rhinitis or conjunctivitis in animal's Intra-nasal administration in an anesthetized animal is easily taught and simple to execute. To order to minimize sneezing, rhinitis and epistaxis, the medications delivered through this pathway should be non-irritating. Mucous membrane of the nasal cavity is rich in blood vessels that can achieve rapid drug absorption and eventual systemic impact, avoiding the initial hepatic-pass effect, which is prominent with the oral administration. Blood levels of intranasally administered drugs may approach the administration intravenously, as these are taken up more quickly through this route due to their tiny and lipophilic molecular nature as compared to those that are of high molecular weight or high polarity.[32, 33]

v. Administration via Inhalational Route

Administration by inhalation apparently uses vapors or either nebulized particles called aerosols in solution. Inhalation usually uses vapors (for example, volatile anesthetic gasses) or solvent aerosols of nebulized particles. With this delivery method, animals are aware and are constrained to enhance delivery with or without a special nose mask. Gravity sedimentation, inertial impaction or diffusion deposits substances administered by aerosol. The alveoli permeate particles less than 3 μm in diameter, and those between 3 and 5 μm in diameter spread evenly across the entire lung. In the mouth through mucociliary apparatus materials are transported up to the trachea after their deposition in the oropharynx, proximal trachea, or airways and then swallowed after absorption by the hepatic first pass mechanisim. The administration of substances through inhalation is a highly complicated technique necessitating specific equipment and understanding. Non-irritating agents should be used to mitigate pharyngeal edema, bronchial spasm, anaphylaxis, per-acute mortality and chronic pulmonary fibrosis. Until beginning the trial, animals should always be conditioned for restraint devices and nasal masks.[34]

General Guidelines for the Administration of Drugs

Maternal rejection of neonatal animals which receive experimental manipulation may be possible. Significant strategies for mitigating dismissal and cannibalism include using gloves to conceal the odors of hands and making sure they treat all young in a litter and making sure the pups are warmed up before being returned to their dams.[35] When special care is taken in the use of quantities of the scale, type and route neonatal animals may be dosed at an early stage. The neonatal strain associated with maternal isolation for testing purposes can significantly influence behavioral indices in the future.[36] Since they grow rapidly, precise body weights are critical before substances are administered. Oral gavage can be given in rodents already after day 1 after birth, although it is more common to wait until after day 4 after birth.[37] The esophageal tissues of neonates are very fine and proper equipment and technique must be used. A 30 gauge needle fixed to a scale of 10 polyethylene tubes is usually used for oral gavage of the rodent pups. Lubed end and a small portion (up to 10 per cent) food color, in order to allow an instant visualization of the substance (via body wall) within the stomach, can be added to the content to be gavaged (typically 0.05 mL for mouse pups).[38] At postnatal day 3 intravenous injections for rodents can begin and the extrinsic jugular and superficial temporal veins can be easily and quickly reachable location.[39] Intraperitoneal and subcutaneous injections are possible given early but due to their limited abdominal capacitance, careful attention to volume is required and intraperitoneal injections are more difficult. The control of annoying substances or large amounts resulting in pain will greatly influence the outcome of the study as either or both these properties may impact the pup's dietary actions leading to the dumping of their feed. In several animals, dams chew and consume the urine and feces of their litters and the impact on the dam of any test material or metabolites excreted by pups should be considered.[40]

Conclusion

Most research experiments are mainly based on the handling of substances by animals. Veterinarians, an animal caregivers from institutions and members of the animal ethics committee need to be considered for proper planning and conducting of studies involving the experimental administration of materials to animals. A close look at the specifics and the mechanism of action will help to improve experiments and minimize harmful effects on animals.

REFERENCES

1. CCAC (The Canadian Council on Animal Care) (2002). Guidelines on Antibody Production, pp. 1–40. CCAC, Ottawa.
2. Donovan, J. and Brown, P. (1991). In Current Protocol in Immunology (eds Coligan *et al.*) pp. 1.4.1–1.4.4. John Wiley and Sons, New York.
3. Woodard, G. (1965). In Methods of Animal Experimentation, Vol. 1 (ed. W.J. Gay), pp. 343–359. Academic Press, NewYork.
4. Waynforth, H. B. and Flecknell, P. A. (1992). In Experimental and Surgical Technique in the Rat (eds H. B. Waynforth and P. A. Flecknell), pp. 1–67. Academic Press, London.
5. Reeves, J.P., Reeves, P.A. and Chin, L.T. (1991). In Current Protocol in Immunology (eds. Coligan *et al.*), pp. 1.6.1–1.6.9. John Wiley and Sons, New York.
6. Food and Drug Administration. [Internet]. 2009. Draft guidance for industry. Animal models: essential elements to address efficacy under the animal rule. Center for Drug Evaluation Research (CDER). [Cited May 2010]. Available at: http: //www.fda.gov/cder/guidance/index.htm.
7. Levine, R.R. (1970). Am. J. Dig. Dis. 15, 171–188.
8. Brady AG. 2000. Research techniques for the squirrel monkey (*Saimiri* spp.). *ILAR J* 41: 10–18.
9. Rosen LB. 2011. Nasogastric tube placement in rabbits. *J Exot Pet Med* 20: 27–31.
10. Cinelli P, Rettich A, Seifert B, Bürki K, Arras M. 2007. Comparative analysis and physiological impact of different tissue biopsy methodologies used for the genotyping of laboratory mice. *Lab Anim* 41: 174–184.
11. The Guide for the Care and Use of Laboratory Animals. NCR. ILAR. Eighth Ed. 2011. P.31.
12. Abe C, Tashiro T, Tanaka K, Ogihara R, Morita HJ. 2009. A novel type of implantable and programmable infusion pump for small laboratory animals. *J Pharmacol Toxicol Methods* 59: 7–12.
13. Eagle CC, Capes DF. 1993. Use of a new syringe pump (Springfusor) for muscle relaxant infusion. *Anaesth Intensive Care* 21: 444–446.

14. Sen S, Chini EN, Brown MJ. 2005. Complications after unintentional intra-arterial injection of drugs: risks, outcomes, and management strategies. *Mayo Clin Proc* 80: 783–795.

15. Sintenie JB, Tuinebreijer WE, Kreis RW, Breederveld RS. 1992. Digital gangrene after accidental intra-arterial injection of phenytoin (epanutin). *Eur J Surg* 158: 315–316.

16. Dubé C, Dubois I, Struthers J. 2011. Intravenous and intraosseous fluid therapy in critically ill birds of prey. *J Exot Pet Med* 20: 21–26.

17. Tobias JD, Kinder Ross A. 2010. Intraosseous infusions: a review for the anesthesiologist with a focus on pediatric use. *Anesth Analg* 110: 391–401.

18. Amin K, Dannenfelser R-M. 2006. *In vitro* hemolysis: guidance for the pharmaceutical scientist. *J Pharm Sci* 95: 1173–1176.

19. Nornoo AO, Osborne DW, Chow DSL. 2008. Cremophor-free intravenous microemulsions for paclitaxel: I: formulation, cytotoxicity, and hemolysis. *Int J Pharm* 349: 108–116.

20. Mazzaferro EM. 2008. Complications of fluid therapy. *Vet Clin North Am Small Anim Pract* 38: 607–619.

21. Ngo MA, Maibach HI. 2010. Dermatotoxicology: historical perspective and advances. *Toxicol Appl Pharmacol* 243: 225–238.

22. Hahn IH, Hoffman RS, Nelson LS. 2004. EMLA-induced methemoglobinemia and systemic topical anesthetic toxicity. *J Emerg Med* 26: 85–88.

23. Ball AM, Smith KM. 2008. Optimizing transdermal drug delivery. *Am J Health Syst Pharm* 65: 1337–1346.

24. Guy RH. 2010. Transdermal drug delivery. *Handb Exp Pharmacol* 197: 399–410.

25. Kagan L, Gershkovich P, Mendelman A, Amsili S, Ezov N, Hoffman A. 2007. The role of the lymphatic system in subcutaneous absorption of macromolecules in the rat model. *Eur J Pharm Biopharm* 67: 759–765.

26. Rasmussen F. 1978. Tissue damage at the injection site after intramuscular injection of drugs. *Vet Res Commun* 2: 173–182.

27. Valverde A. 2008. Epidural analgesia and anesthesia in dogs and cats. *Vet Clin North Am Sm Anim Pract* 38: 1205–1230.

28. Lukas G, Brindle SD, Greengard P. 1971. The route of absorption of intraperitoneally administered compounds. *J Pharmacol Exp Ther* 178: 562–566.

29. Coria-Avila GA, Gavrila AM, Ménard S, Ismail N, Pfaus JG. 2007. Cecum location in rats and the implications for intraperitoneal injections. *Lab Anim (NY)* 36: 25–30.

30. Gotloib L, Wajsbrot V, Shostak A. 2005. A short review of experimental peritoneal sclerosis: from mice to men. *Int J Artif Organs* 28: 97–104.

31. Vachon P, Faubert S, Blais D, Comtois A, Bienvenu JG. 2000. A pathophysiological study of abdominal organs following intraperitoneal injections of chloral

hydrate in rats: comparison between two anesthesia protocols. *Lab Anim* 34: 84–90.

32. Hall LW, Clarke KW, Trim CM, editors. 2001. Veterinary anesthesia, 10th ed. Philadelphia (PA): Saunders.
33. Illum L. 2002. Nasal drug delivery: new developments and strategies. *Drug Discov Today* 7: 1184–1189.
34. Pauwels R, Newman S, Borgström L. 1997. Airway deposition and airway effects of antiasthma drugs delivered from metered-dose inhalers. *Eur Respir J* 10: 2127–2138.
35. Lipman NS, Newcomer CE, Fox JG. 1987. Rederivation of MHV and MEV antibody positive mice by cross-fostering and use of the microisolator caging system. *Lab Anim Sci* 37: 195–199.
36. Lu L, Mamiya T, Lu P, Niwa M, Mouri A, Zou LB, Nagai T, Hiramatsu M, Nabeshima T. 2009. The long-lasting effects of cross-fostering on the emotional behavior in ICR mice. *Behav Brain Res* 198: 172–178.
37. Moser VC, Walls I, Zoetis T. 2005. Direct dosing of preweaning rodents in toxicity testing and research: deliberations of an ILSI RSI expert working group. *Int J Toxicol* 24: 87–94.
38. Ramig RF. 1988. The effects of host age, virus dose, and virus strain on heterologous rotavirus infection of suckling mice. *Microb Pathog* 4: 189–202.
39. Kienstra KA, Freysdottir D, Gonzales NM, Hirsch KK. 2007. Murine neonatal intravascular injections: modeling newborn disease. *J Am Assoc Lab Anim Sci* 46: 50–54.
40. Biesemeier JA, Beck MJ, Silberberg H, Myers NR, Ariano JM, Bodle ES, Sved DW, Jacobi S, Stump DG, Hardy M, Stedeford T. 2010. Effects of dose, administration route, and/or vehicle on decabromodiphenyl ether concentrations in plasma of maternal, fetal, and neonatal rats and in milk of maternal rats. *Drug Metab Dispos* 38: 1648–1654.

Chapter 2

Methods of Collection of Blood from Laboratory Animals

Blood collection from small laboratory animals is necessary for a broad range of scientific research and there are various efficient methods available for that. Hence, it is important that blood sample collection from experimental animals should be stressful because stress will affect the result[1]. So there are various guidelines which we follow for blood collection in laboratory animal approved by the Institute animal ethics committee.

- It should be least stressful and painful and collected with or without anesthesia[2].
- Adequate training is required for blood collection using any method in any species. Restrain is also necessary to prevent movement that may result in laceration of blood vessels or other organs or serious complications. It should be chosen based on species.
- The volume and method of blood to be collected will depend on various factors like animal species, frequency of collection, and experimental needs. So, one should plan the protocol and perform it with an appreciation for the stresses associated with loss of blood to the animal and do whatever that can minimize the animal's reaction to the stress. Careful planning and control of blood sampling and all experimental variables associated with it should not only benefit the welfare of the animal but also minimize confounding influences on research data[3].
- The frequency of blood collection is important. Once in two weeks is ideal for non-rodents. If the study needs multiple blood samples, lagomorphs (*e.g.*, hares and rabbits) can be used.

- If the study involves repeated blood sample collection, the samples can be withdrawn through a temporary cannula. This may reduce pain and stress in the experimental animals.
- Collection of blood by tail vessels or lacerating an ear required approval from IACUC. There is chances of lacerating an artery rather than vein resulting in severe haemorrhage; in addition, these methods are more painful than needle puncture because of prolonged time for wound healing and sometimes it further leads to various other complications.
- An animal may not be returned to its cage until complete homeostasis has been achieved.

If too much blood is drawn too quickly or too frequently without replacement, animals may develop hypovolemic shock. In the longer term, the removal of too much blood causes anemia, muscle weakness, increased susceptibility to cold, and reduced exercise tolerance. If 15 per cent to 20 per cent of the blood volume is removed, cardiac output and blood pressure will be reduced. Removal of 30 per cent to 40 per cent can induce shock and death. It is extremely important to apply pressure to the blood collection site, especially when penetrating an artery, for at least 3 to 5 minutes post blood collection to prevent hematoma formation. The Animal Care Services (ACS) limits survival blood collection to 10 per cent of the animal's circulating blood volume. The frequency of blood collection is dependent upon the volume collected. If the maximum volume, as specified above, is collected within a 24 hour period, blood may be collected once every two weeks. The monitoring of hematocrit, serum protein levels, and potentially replacement fluid therapy is indicated when more frequent and/or higher volume collections are scientifically necessary; however, scientific justification is required[8].

Single Blood Draw

A maximum of 1 per cent of body weight can be removed as single blood draw every 14 days, without requiring administration of supplemental replacement fluids. Withdrawing the minimum amount of blood necessary is strongly recommended. Examples:

- 0.15 ml from a 15 g mouse
- 3 ml from a 300 g rat
- 30 ml from a 3 kg rabbit

Multiple Blood Draws

If the total volume withdrawn over a 14 day period is less than 1 per cent BW, then no additional action needs to be taken. If the total volume withdrawn over a 14 day period is up to 2 per cent BW, fluid volume replacement must be considered. Withdrawing the minimum amount of blood necessary is strongly recommended. Examples:

- Up to 0.15 ml withdrawn from a 15 g mouse over 2 weeks is OK

- Up to 0.3 ml withdrawn from a 15 g mouse over 2 weeks, replace volume with 0.3 ml saline SC
- Up to 3 ml from a 300 g rat over 2 weeks is OK
- Up to 6 ml from a 300 g rat over 2 weeks, replace volume with 6 ml saline SC
- Up to 30 ml from a 3 kg rabbit over 2 weeks is OK
- Up to 60 ml from a 3 kg rabbit over 2 weeks, replace volume with 60 ml saline SC

As a helpful guideline, daily blood draws under 0.07 per cent BW will keep the total 2-week withdrawal under 1 per cent BW.

Recommended Blood Collection Volumes are Intended to Preserve the Health Status of the Animal and Maintain the Validity of Experimental Results

Species	*Blood Volume (ml/kg)*
Mouse	72
Rat	64
Guinea pig	75
Hamster	78
Rabbit	65
Ferret	70

Blood Collections Site

Species	*Recommended sites*
Mouse	Lateral tail veins puncture, saphenous vein,orbital venous sinus requires anesthesia, cardiac puncture under anesthesia and amputation of tail tip
Rat	Lateral Tail vein, saphenous vein, sublingual veins, dorsal pedal vein, orbital venous sinus requires anesthesia and cardiac puncture under anesthesia.
Guinea pig	Lateral sephanous or tarsal vein, ear vein, Juglar vein, cardiac puncture
Hamster	jugular vein, the tail vein, the saphenous vein, orbital venous sinus, cardiac puncture and cephalic vein
Rabbit	*Marginal ear vein, central ear artery, sephanous vein and Cardiac puncture (diaphragmatic approach) jugular vein*
Ferret	Lateral saphenous, cephalic vein jugular vein and cranial vena cava

MOUSE

1. Lateral Tail Vein Puncture

The tail vein blood collection is suitable for all strains of mice, and it is quick and simple to perform. However, prior to this technique the mice, need to be warmed so as to dilate the blood vessel. The lateral tail vein is located on the lateral aspect of the mouse's tail. A needle size of 23- 25 gauge can be used for 1 ml of blood. The use of a needle without a syringe, allowing the hub to fill with blood, and subsequent collection into a microhematocrit tube is useful when very small quantities of blood are needed. The blood sample should be collected from the distal end first and then moving towards the proximal end; since taking the first sample from the proximal end of the tail can cause a perivascular clot and inflammation than can significantly reduce the blood flow to the distal portion of the blood vessel (NCRRRAR, 2017; Johns Hopkins University, 2017)

2. Saphenous Vein

The blood sample is taken from the saphenous vein, which runs dorsally and laterally over the tarsal joint. The site is first shaved (hairs removed). The mice should be restrained. The hind limb should be immobilized in the extended position prior to blood collection. If the animal is difficult to handle, mild anesthesia should be given to the animal. A puncture is made with the help of fine needle to collect the blood sample. The number of attempts to puncture the vein should not exceed three in one attempt. Blood flow can be stopped by pressing gently with a finger above the puncture site and the animal should only be returned to the cage after the blood flow has stopped completely[2].

3. Orbital Venous Sinus Collection

The sinus surrounding the globe of the mouse's eye is a useful site for collecting larger volumes of blood. General anesthesia must be provided when collecting from this site. Under general anesthesia the mouse is grasped so that its back rests on the palm of your left hand (right hand if you are left-handed) with its head toward your thumb. The thumb is placed just lateral to the animal's trachea so that the jugular vein on the same side as the eye from which you are collecting blood is occluded and the fur on the animals head is drawn into the palm of your hand. This causes the animal's eye to proptose (bulge) slightly. Be careful not to occlude the trachea! A 50 uL sterile microhematocrit tube is directed into the medial canthus (junction of eyelids closest to the animal's nose) of the eye rotating slightly as the tube is directed to a point directly behind the globe. Sufficient pressure must be applied to cut through the fibrous layer that surrounds the sinus. Blood flows through the tube and occasionally around the tube once the sinus has been penetrated. After blood collection, the tube is removed and the eyelids closed and a dry cotton pad is applied over the eye with gentle pressure to prevent retro orbital hemorrhage. In general blood should not be collected from the same eye more than 2 times, allowing at least 2 weeks between collections. An antibiotic ophthalmic ointment must be applied following bleeding.

The orbital venous sinus route has been commonly used by researchers in the past but has been observed to cause many adverse effects i) retro orbital hemorrhage resulting in hematoma and excessive pressure on the eye, which is almost certainly painful for the animal; (ii) any pressure required to stem persistent bleeding (*e.g.* by pressing on the eye) or pressure from a hematoma can lead to corneal ulceration, keratitis, pannus formation, rupture of the globe and micro-ophthalmia; (iii) damage to the optic nerve and other intra-orbital structures, which can lead to deficits in vision and even blindness; (iv) fracture of the fragile bones of the orbit and neural damage by the micropipette.

4. Cardiac Puncture (Diaphragmatic Approach)

Cardiac puncture is the preferred technique for the terminal collection of large blood volumes. General anesthesia must be administered and the animal placed on its back on a solid surface. The xiphoid process is palpated at the caudal aspect of the animal's sternum. A notch is present on both sides of this process. A 1 inch 22 or higher gauge needle attached to a 1 - 3 mL syringe is inserted into either notch and directed toward the heart as determined by palpating for the heartbeat. Once the needle has been inserted beneath the skin, gentle negative pressure should be applied by pulling backward on the plunger. The animal must be sacrificed at the completion of the procedure prior to awakening from anesthesia.

5. Amputation of the Tail Tip

This technique is commonly used in mice, with sample volumes of 0.1–0.2 mL being obtained. Amputation should be restricted to the tail tip (0.5–1 mm should be adequate, and over time only a maximum of 5 mm can be removed). Repeat bleeding is feasible in the short term by removing the clot. Serial amputations resulting in a significant shortening of the tail (>5 mm) are not acceptable. The technique may not be suitable for older animals. Anesthesia is required for any mice 3 weeks old or older[3].

RAT

1. Lateral Tail Vein Puncture

The procedure for collecting blood from the rat's tail vein is similar to the technique described for the mouse. A slightly larger gauge needle (24 gauge) can be utilized. Because of the vein's size, larger blood volumes (approximately 1 mL)

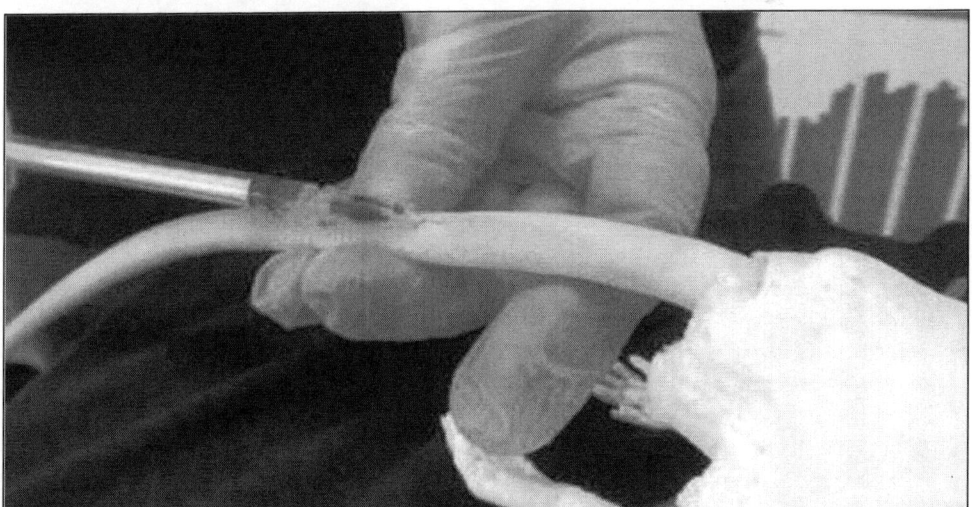

Figure 2.1: Blood Collection from Lateral Tail Vein Puncture.

may be obtained from adult rats. As for mice, for small blood volume collection, the tail vein can be simply punctured with a small gauge needle. Free flowing drops of blood can be collected, as with the facial or saphenous vein techniques.

2. Saphenous Vein

Blood sample collection from the lateral saphenous vein is a relatively quick method of blood collection from all strains of rats. This technique does not require the rat to be anesthetized. In blood sample collection procedure is the same as discussed in mice.The site is first shaved (hairs removed). The rat should be restrained. This may stress the rat; herefore, the duration of restraint should be as minimum as possible. The hind limb should be immobilized in the extended position prior to blood collection. If the animal is difficult to handle mild anesthesia should be given to the animal. A puncture is made with the help of fine needle to collect the blood sample. The number of attempts to puncture the vein should not exceed three in one attempt. Blood flow can be stopped by pressing gently with a finger above the puncture site, and the animal should only be returned to the cage after the blood flow has stopped completely[6].

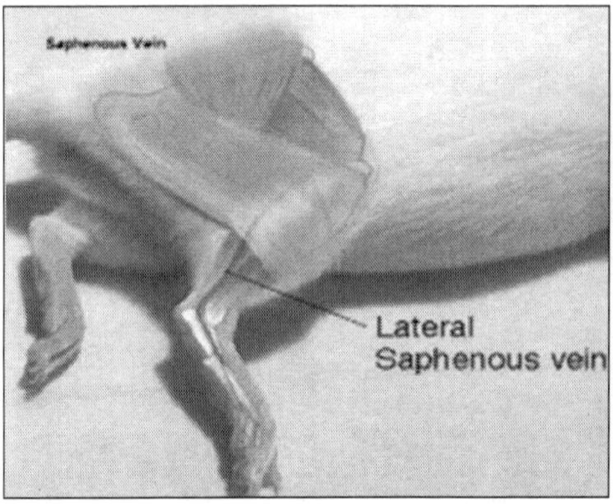

Figure 2.2: Blue Color Indicate Lateral Saphenous Vein (Lateral view).

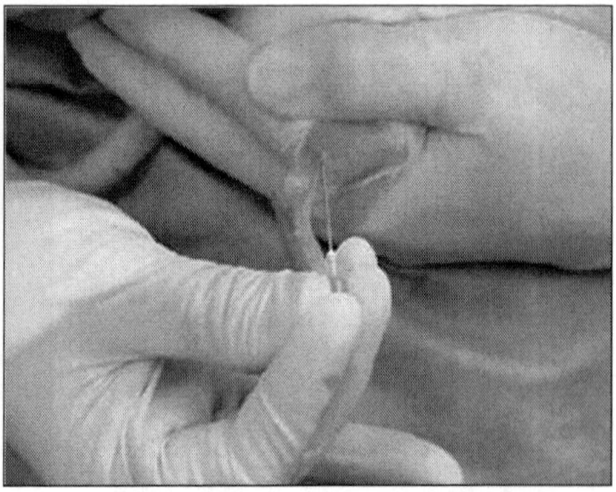

Figure 2.3: Blood Collection from Saphenous Vein.

3. Sublingual Vein

This technique is easy to perform in rats and is suitable for the removal of large volumes of blood (*e.g.* 0.2–1 ml) at frequent intervals, limited only by the blood volume to be removed and by the necessarily repeated anesthesia. A refined method avoids some of the disadvantages previously seen and can be used for repeated sampling. Rats are anesthetized and held by an assistant in a supine position. The loose skin at the nape of the neck is gathered up in order to produce partial stasis in the venous return from the head. A second person gently pulls out the tongue with a cotton-tipped applicator stick, grasps it with thumb and forefinger and one of the sublingual veins (there is one on each side of the midline) is punctured with a 23–25 g hypodermic needle as near to the tip of the tongue as possible. The rat is turned over to allow blood to drip into a tube and after the requisite volume of blood has been obtained the compression at the scruff of the neck is released and the animal is placed in a supine position. The tongue is again extended in order to stem the flow of blood with a dry cotton-tipped applicator stick; usually there is no need to use any haemostatic agent. With this technique, rats do not show any significant differences in food or water consumption or body weight gain compared with untreated anesthetized control animals.

4. Dorsal Pedal Vein

The rat is restrained, and the hind food around the ankle is held, and the medial dorsal pedal vessel is located. The foot is cleaned with absolute alcohol and the vein is punctured with a fine needle. The blood will start dropping out. The blood drops are collected in a capillary tube.

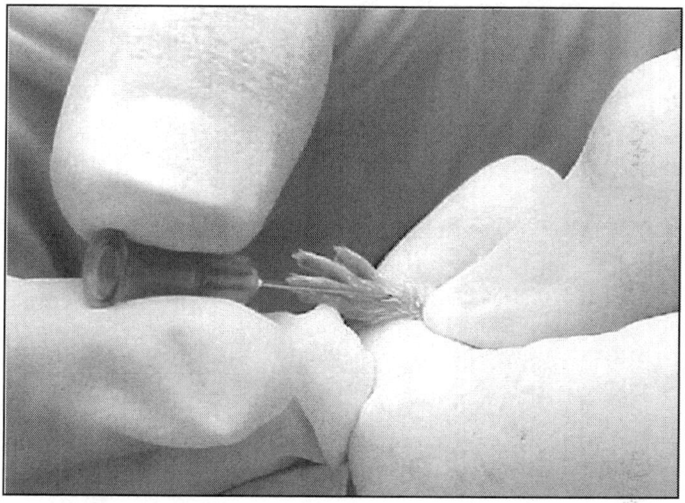

Figure 2.4: Blood Collection from Dorsal Pedal Vein.

5. Orbital Venous Sinus

For this technique, the rat needs to be anesthetized and the method is the same as discussed above in mice.

6. Cardiac Puncture

The cardiac puncture blood collection technique is recommended for terminal stage of the study to collect a single, good quality volume of blood from the animals. The blood sample is taken from the heart, from the ventricle slowly to avoid collapsing of the heart. A 23G1 needle may be used. The rat is deeply anesthetized. To ensure prolonged anesthesia, a paper towel soaked in volatile anesthetic is placed on rat's nose during the procedure. The rat is placed on its back. Place your finger at the level of lowest ribs without applying any pressure. The heart is roughly 1

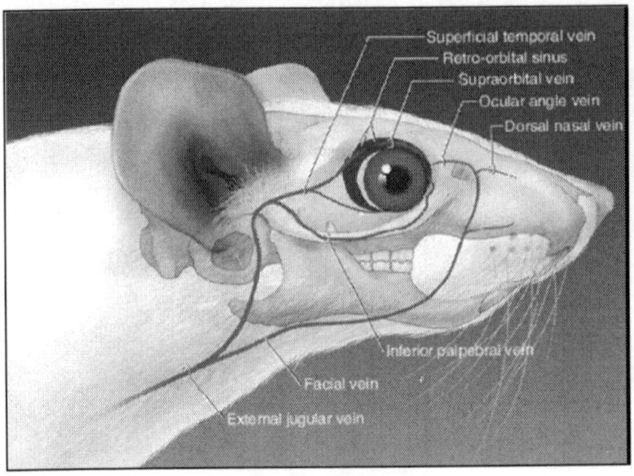

Figure 2.5: Position of Orbital Sinus.

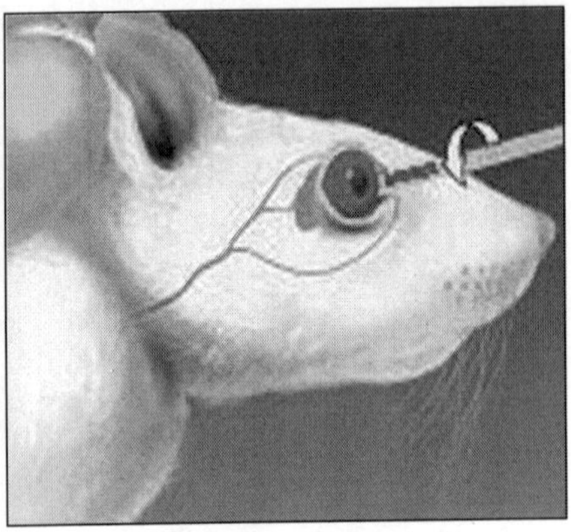

Figure 2.6: Blood Collection from Orbital Sinus.

cm above this point, slightly right. Now holding the syringe at 45 degree angle, the needle is inserted between the two ribs and watched for a drop of blood which ascertains that the needle is inside the heart. Without moving the syringe, the syringe plunger is pulled to fill the syringe with blood. Once the syringe is full, it is carefully disconnected from the needle and emptied into a tube. The syringe can then be reattached to collect more blood, and it is possible to draw 5-10 ml of blood from 150-200 gm rat. The rat should be immediately euthanized post blood collection.

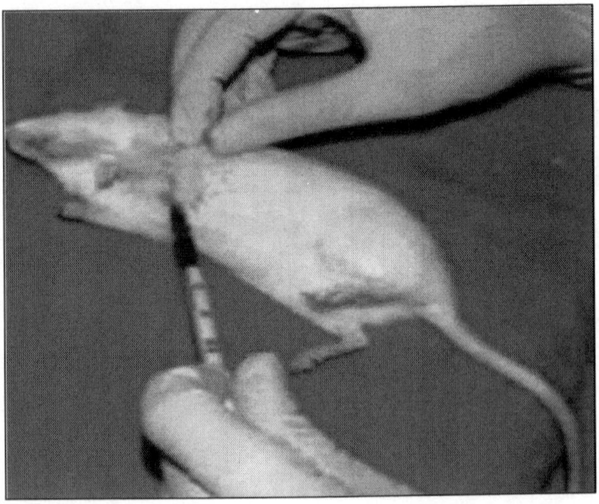

Figure 2.7: Blood collection from Cardiac Puncture.

GUINEA PIGS

1. Lateral Saphenous or Tarsal Vein

Perform this procedure without anesthesia and the help of one investigator, one handling the guinea pig, and one collecting the sample. Shave the tarsal region of the hind leg with an electric shaver until the veins are visible. Ensure the area is large enough to avoid fur interfering with the puncture site. Place the hind leg in a lukewarm water bath and gently rub the leg, making the veins more dilated and evident. Wipe the leg with a clean towel and disinfect the puncture site with gauze or a cotton swab dampened with 70 per cent alcohol. Restrain the guinea pig and extend the hind leg downward while applying gentle pressure immediately above the knee joint to provide stasis. Puncture the vein using a 21 G needle or lancet. Collect blood *e.g.*, by using a collection or capillary tube. Gently manipulate the leg to aid the blood flow. Release stasis, once the sample has been obtained. Apply a piece of gauze or cotton wool with gentle pressure to the puncture site until bleeding has stopped. Return the animal to its cage and monitor for 5-10 min to ensure hemostasis[7].

2. Ear Vein

This procedure is also without anesthesia either alone or preferably with the help of one colleague. **Firstly** disinfect the dorsal surface of the ear using gauze or a cotton swab dampened with 70 per cent alcohol. **Then** apply light pressure to the base of the ear to provide stasis. Puncture the vein using a 21 G needle or lancet, and collect blood. Release stasis, once the sample has been obtained, Apply a piece of gauze or cotton wool with gentle pressure to the puncture site until bleeding has stopped. Return the animal to its cage and monitor for 5-10 min to ensure hemostasis.

3. Jugular Vein

Carry out this procedure using the help of one additional investigator; one handling the guinea pig and one collecting the sample. Anesthetize the guinea pig with a suitable anesthetic for the entire duration of this procedure. A mixture of tiletamine (0.93 mg/kg), zolazepam (0.93 mg/kg), xylazine (1.49 mg/kg) and butorphanol (0.06 mg/kg) can be used.

Place the anesthetized guinea pig on its back and gently retract the forelegs caudally. Shave and disinfect (*e.g.*, with 70 per cent alcohol) the ventral part of the neck. Coat the syringe with either heparin or EDTA prior to sampling in order to reduce the risk of clotting. Palpate the clavicle and insert a 25 G (or 23 G) needle mounted on a 1 ml syringe approximately 1 cm lateral to the midline at the level of the shoulder joint. Keep the syringe in a slight upward and medial angle while applying slight negative pressure. Avoid damaging the underlying structures as the jugular vein is situated quite superficial. Tilt the neck of the guinea pig slightly backward to provide increased stasis of the vein. Release the front legs when the blood sample is obtained, and alleviate stasis before the needle is retracted. Use a dry piece of gauze or cotton wool to apply gentle pressure to the puncture site. Return the animal to a recovery cage and monitor to ensure hemostasis and recovery from anesthesia[3].

4. Cardiac Puncture (Terminal Procedure)

The technique for cardiac puncture from the guinea pig is identical to that described for mice. This procedure is performed as a terminal event only and general anesthesia is required. The animal must be sacrificed at the completion of the procedure prior to awakening from anesthesia.

HAMSTER

There are various acceptable blood collection sites/methods for the hamster. These include the jugular vein, the tail vein, the cephalic vein, and the saphenous vein, and these are discussed earlier and in addition to those described below[14].

1. Orbital Venous Sinus

This technique is not recommended.The technique describing blood collection from the mouse's orbital venous sinus should be followed for orbital venous sinus collection in the hamster except the microhematocrit tube should be inserted into the lateral canthus rather than the medial. The technique must be performed under general anesthesia and post-bleeding hemostasis is essential to prevent complications.

2. Cardiac Puncture (Terminal Procedure)

The technique for cardiac puncture from the hamster is identical to that described for the mouse. A 22 gauge needle is recommended. A 3 - 5 cc syringe should be used if large blood volumes are desired. This procedure is performed under general anesthesia as a terminal event only. The animal must be sacrificed at the completion of the procedure prior to awakening from anesthesia.

3. Lateral Saphenous Vein

The approach to the hamster's lateral saphenous vein is similar to the mouse, but a 20- to 25-gauge needle is used to collect the blood.

4. Cephalic Vein

The hamster should be placed under general anesthesia when collecting blood from the cephalic vein. A tourniquet should be placed around the leg proximal to the elbow. The approach to the cephalic vein is similar to that of the cat, although a 25-gauge needle is inserted into the vein and the blood is collected from the hub of the needle.

RABBIT

The marginal ear vein and central ear artery are useful sites for the collection of moderate volumes of blood from rabbits that are to survive the procedure. Vasodilatation can be induced by administering a phenothiazine tranquilizer and alpha adrenergic receptor blocker (acepromazine) at least 5 - 10 minutes, up to one hour, prior to blood collection. A 21G or higher gauge butterfly needle is recommended. The insertion site is disinfected using an alcohol soaked pad prior to inserting the needle, bevel up, into the artery or vein. After the blood collection, it is essential to apply pressure to the artery over the insertion site for at least 3 minutes to provide suitable haemostasis. Significant blood loss can occur from the artery in particular, if adequate haemostasis is not provided[4].

1. Marginal Ear Vein

Place the rabbit in a rabbit restrainer. Using clippers, remove the hair from the ear. Place a finger, loosely fitting paper clip, or an other form of light tourniquet at the base of the ear. Use a 25-gauge, 5/8-inch, or 22-gauge, 1-inch needle. Small quantities can be collected from the hub of a 25-gauge needle directly into a microhematocrit tube. The larger needle is attached to a syringe and blood is collected slowly into the syringe to avoid collapsing the vein. If blood does not flow readily, there may be a clot formation in the needle or too much negative pressure applied to the syringe. Release the negative pressure and slowly rotate the needle. Repeat these steps as needed until the desired quantity of blood has been collected.

A tranquilizer, such as Innovar-Vet or Ace-Promazine, works very well as a vasodilator as well as providing a tranquilizing effect. Administer Innovar-Vet at a dose of 0.1 to 0.2 ml per rabbit SQ or IM; or Ace-Promazine 0.25 to 0.5 mg/kg SQ or IM. The best results are obtained when administered 10-15 minutes prior to blood collection.

2. Central Ear Artery

Place the rabbit in a rabbit restrainer. Using clippers, remove the hair from the ear. A 1 to 1-1/2-inch needle ranging in size from 22-gauge to 20-gauge is recommended for blood collection. Some investigators prefer to break off the hub of the needle and use the needle shaft for collection or to use a vaccutainer needle. Extend the ear away from the rabbit's head to provide a flat surface and insert the needle into the artery. Once blood begins to flow, lower the ear and position the receptacle under the needle for blood collection. Occasionally, the artery may constrict during the collection process, shutting off the flow of blood. Hold the needle securely in place until the rabbit relaxes, usually within one minute. Gentle massage of the artery at the base of the ear may enhance blood flow. Clot formation in the needle can also prevent blood flow. If no blood flows, remove the needle and repeat the procedure using a new needle. Insert the new needle into the artery proximal to the previous site (closer to the base of the ear).

3. Saphenous Vein

An attendant restrains the rabbit, exposing the rear leg to the person drawing the specimen. Hair is clipped from the lateral saphenous vein on the lower rear limb. The vein is occluded by the attendant and the phlebotomist cleans and dries the skin over the vein with alcohol and sterile gauze. Using a scalp vein set primed with sodium heparin, a 21-24 gauge needle is inserted into the occluded vessel and blood is aspirated into the connected 3 ml syringe prefilled with 1 ml of air.

4. Cardiac Puncture (Diaphragmatic Approach)

Large volumes of blood can be collected directly from the heart of anesthetized rabbits as a terminal event. The technique is similar to that described for mice and rats, however, a larger needle and syringe (1.5in >18 gauge; >20 cc) should be used.

5. Jugular Vein

Under general anesthesia for jugular venipuncture in rabbits. However, if the animal is calm, it can be wrapped in a towel or a cat bag for restraint. The biggest concern associated with jugular venipuncture is compromising the animal's breathing when its head is extended. To limit the likelihood of problems, the animal's breathing should be monitored closely during the procedure. When a rabbit is in sternal recumbence, the approach to jugular venipuncture is similar to that of a cat. Jugular venipuncture can be difficult in obese animals or in does with a large dewlap. In cases where the dewlap is in the way, it can be displaced ventrally with the phlebotomist's thumb to help gain access to the jugular vein. A rabbit can also be placed in dorsal recumbence with its head extended for sample collection. The jugular vein can be approached from a cranio caudal or caudo cranial direction in relation to the head[15].

FERRET

1. Lateral Saphenous Vein

To collect blood from a ferret's lateral saphenous vein, the animal should be placed in ventral or lateral recumbency and the rear leg grasped just distal to the stifle to engorge the vessel. A 26- to 27-gauge needle on a 1-mL syringe can be used to decrease the risk of vessel collapse during the blood draw. A topical anesthetic cream should be applied to the vessel 30 minutes before sample collection to minimize patient discomfort.

2. Cephalic Vein

The ferret can be wrapped in a towel for restraint or grasped by the scruff of the neck and held in a vertical position. By restraining the patient's "scruff," the animal becomes passive and will allow the foreleg to be held and a tourniquet placed above the elbow.47 A topical anesthetic cream should be applied 30 minutes before this procedure. For cephalic venipuncture, a 25- to 26-gauge needle on a 1-mL syringe is recommended.

3. Jugular Vein

A 20- to 25-gauge needle should be used to collect the sample, and bending the needle at a 30° angle will help facilitate sample collection. The animal can be wrapped in a towel or restrained with the head and neck extended and the forelegs pulled down over the edge of the table. Shaving the fur over the vein and applying pressure at the thoracic inlet will help the phlebotomist visualize the vein. Isoflurane anesthesia can be used to help facilitate sample collection from fractious animals.

4. Cranial Vena Cava

Ferrets have a very long thoracic cavity, and their heart lies in the caudal aspect of their thorax. Because of the caudal location of their heart, the risk of cardiac puncture with cranial vena cava venipuncture in this species is minimal. To access the cranial vena cava of a ferret, the patient should be grasped by the scruff of the neck and placed in dorsal recumbency. The head should be positioned off the edge of the table, keeping the head and neck in alignment with the body, while the front legs are pulled back along the chest. To prevent rotation of the forelegs, two fingers should be placed between the legs. Another person is required to support the body just cranial to the pelvis. It is not necessary to hold the back legs, and this may be stressful to the animal. A 25- to 27-gauge, 0.5-inch needle on a 3-mL syringe can be used for sample collection. The needle should be inserted into the thoracic notch between the manubrium and the sternum, just cranial to the first rib. Minimal negative pressure is required within the syringe as the needle is advanced. If the animal is difficult to handle, general anesthesia should be used for sample collection[10, 11].

REFERENCES

1. Parasuraman S, Raveendran R, Kesavan R. Blood sample collection in small laboratory animals. *J Pharmacol Pharmacother* 2010; **1:** 87-93
2. Hoff J, Rlagt LV. Methods of blood collection in the mouse. Lab animals 2000; 29: 47-53
3. McGuill M.W. and Rowan A.N. Biological Effects of Blood Loss: Implications for Sampling Volumes and Techniques. ILAR News (1989), 31(4): 5-18.
4. Procedure for rabbit blood collection [online]. Available from: http: //www. research.uky.edu/ori/univet/resources/sop/Procedure_rabbit_blood_ collection.pdf [Last cited on 2010 Feb 23].
5. Johns Hopkins University. url: http: //web.jhu.edu/animalcare/procedures/ retro-orbital.html; visited on 06-02-2017; 27: 43 hrs; India
6. National Centre for the Replacement Refinement and Reduction of Animals in Research, url: https: //www.nc3rs.org.uk/rat-saphenous-vein-non-surgical; visited on 05-02-2017; 23: 32 Hrs; India.
7. Abatan Ol, Welch KB, Nemzek JA (2008). Evaluation of saphenous venipunture and modified tail clip blood collection in mice. Journal of the American association for laboratory animal science, 47(3): 8-15.
8. A Good Practice Guide to the Administration of Substances and Removal of Blood, Including Routes and Volumes, Diehl, *et.al.*, Journal of Applied Toxicology, 21, 15–23 (2001)
9. Parasuraman, S., Raveendran, R. and Kesavan, R: Blood sample collection in small laboratory animals. Journal of Pharmacology and Pharmacotherapeutics 1(2): 87 – 93 (2010).
10. Hem, A., Smith, A.J., and Solberg, P. Saphenous vein puncture for blood sampling of the mouse, rat, hamster, gerbil, guinea pig, ferret and mink. *Lab Anim.* **32** (4), 364-368, (1998).
11. Parasuraman, S., Raveendran, R., and Kesavan, R. Blood sample collection in small laboratory animals. *J.Pharmacol.Pharmacother.* **1** (2), 87-93, (2010).

12. Hem A, Smith AJ, Solberg P: Saphenous vein puncture for blood sampling of the mouse, rat, hamster, gerbil, guinea pig, ferret and mink. *Lab Anim* **32**: 364-368, (1998).

13. Timm KI: Orbital venous anatomy of the Mongolian gerbil with comparison to the mouse, hamster and rat. *Lab Anim Sci* **39:** 262-264, 1989.

14. Biomethod for obtaining gastric juice and serum from the unanesthetized guinea pig (*Cavia porcellus*). *Contemp Top Lab Anim Sci* **38**: 32-35, 1999

Chapter 3

Methods for Detection of Antimicrobial Resistance

Introduction

Antibiotics are the antimicrobial substances that are used to destroy or kill the microbes that are causing diseases. The discovery of these wander drugs or magic bullets in the mid 20th century, made the scientists believe that these antibiotics could eliminate disease causing bacteria without causing harmful effects to the host. Alexander Fleming and Paul Ehrlich were the two who led to the beginning of an era of modern antibiotics[1]. Antibiotics work either by killing or by inhibiting the growth of micro-organism thus, facilitate the immune system of host to eliminate the microbes from the body. Mechanism of action of these magic bullets- inhibition of synthesis of bacterial cell, synthesis of proteins, DNA, RNA, or by a membrane disorganizing agent. They also act by binding to the cell wall of bacteria, using energy-dependent transport mechanisms in ribosomal sites, which result into the inhibition of protein synthesis.

Antibiotic resistance or resistome is the inability of antibiotics to eliminating the micro-organism from the host effectively. It is the resistance of micro-organsim towards the action of antibiotics causing havoc in the field of medical sciences and such bacteria are called resistant bacteria which multiply even in the therapeutically presence of antibiotics. Non-judicial use of antibiotics is one of the main reason for the development of antibiotic resistance. Mithicillin resistant *Staphylococcus* aureus (MRSA), vancomycin resistant *Staphylococcus* aureus (VSRA), aminoglycoside-resistant strains of *Staphylococcus* aureus are some examples of antibiotic resistant strains of *Staphylococcus* aureus.

Antimicrobial Resistance

AMR defined as the resistance to all micro-organism towards their respective drugs. When bacteria become resistant to the drug, it requires a higher dose of drug for its elimination from the host than the normal concentration. In 1920, the discovery of Penicillin by Alexander Fleming had bought the revolution in the field of medical sciences. As the discovery of new antibiotics increases with the time, resistance against the antibiotics also gain pace. In Thailand, for treating non-cholera diarrhea, sulphamethoxazole and trimethoprim (TMP-SMZ), ampicillin and tetracycline were used for many years but now due to resistance, have no role in treatment[2].

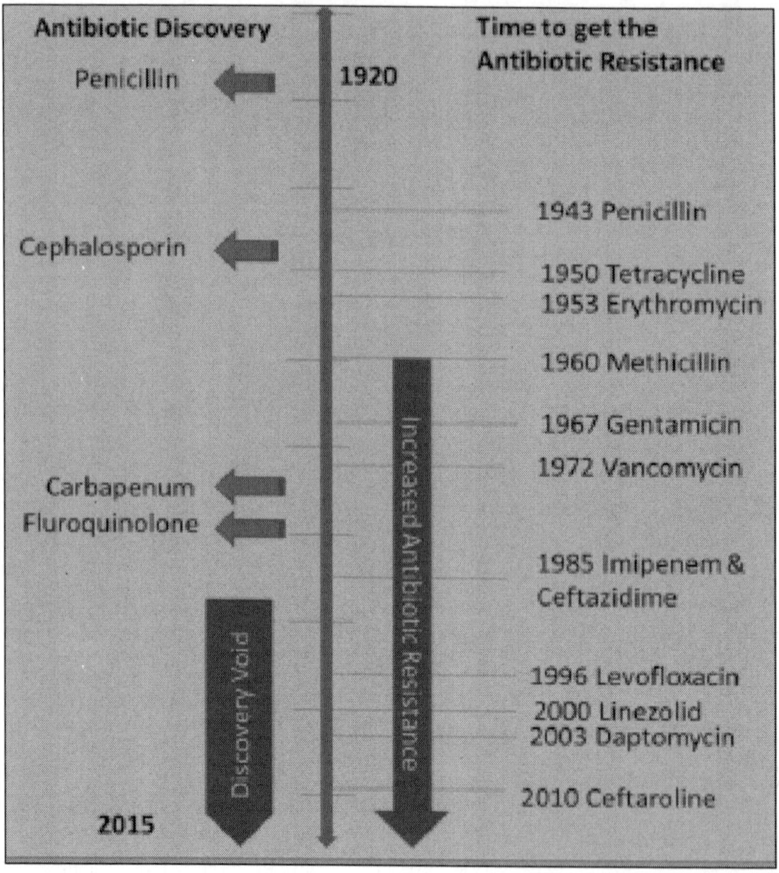

Figure 2.1: Antibiotic Discovery versus Development of Antimicrobial Resistance.

Bacteria resist action of antibiotics through four major mechanism (1) modification of target site, (2) modification or destruction of antibiotic, (3) antibiotic efflux via efflux transporters, (4) reduced antibiotic influx through decreased membrane permeability (Figure 2.2)[2].

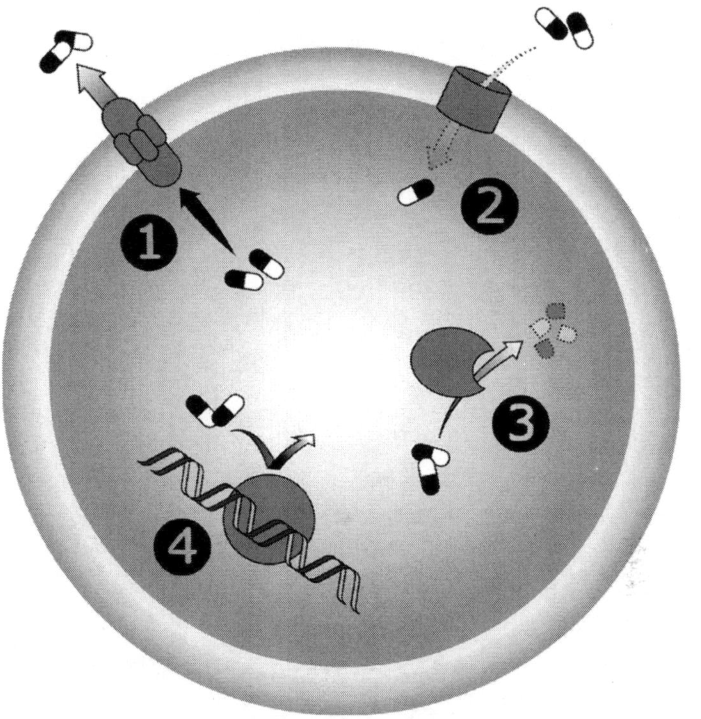

Figure 2.2: Major Molecular Pathways Used by Bacteria to Resist the Mechanism of Action of Antibiotic: (1) increased drug efflux, (2) Decreased drug influx, (3) Destruction/modification of drug, (4) Modification of target site.

Bacteria may acquire the resistance through vertical (endogenous) or horizontal (exogenous) evolution. Endogenous evolution involves the mutation occurring in the genome of bacterium resulting in the resistance while the exogenous evolution carry out by transfering the resistant genes to the susceptible bacteria. Conjugation, transformation and transduction are the methods use by bacteria in horizontal evolution.

Many strategies have been made to combat the antimicrobial resistance so that antibiotics can be effectively uses for the treatment of bacteria, one such strategy is antibiotic resistance breakers (ARBs). These are compounds that enable the host to utilize the antibiotics efficiently by attacking the resistance mechanism employed against antibiotics. ARBs include three major classes : modifying-enzyme inhibitors, membrane permeabilisers and efflux pump inhibitors (EPIs). Modifying-enzyme inhibitors include β-lactamase inhibitors, aminoglycoside- modifying enzyme inhibitors. Membrane permeabilisers include the polymixins.

Determination of Antimicrobial Resistance

AMR is the growing serious threat to the mankind, as it does not allow the antibiotics to destroy the bacteria in the host effectively therefore, it is necessary to identify the resistant bacteria. Testing of AMR can be done through phenotypic and genotypic methods. Phenotypic methods include qualitative and quantitative tests.

Qualitative Tests

1. Disk Diffusion Method

It is the most frequently used method for determining antimicrobial resistance. This test is based on the estimation of the zone of inhibition is proportional to the bacterial susceptibility to the antibiotic present in the disk. Inoculum of about 1-2X108 log CFU/ml of examining micro-organism is applying on the surface of the nutrient agar plate. Antibiotic disk which is to be tested is placed over the nutrient agar plate. Result to be recorded after 24 hrs by measuring the zone of growth inhibition of examined mico-organism[3]. Disk diffusion test is cheap, easy to perform, simple, well-standardized and can be used as a screening test against large number of isolates. On the basis of zone of inhibition, examined micro-organism is categorized as susceptible and resistant.

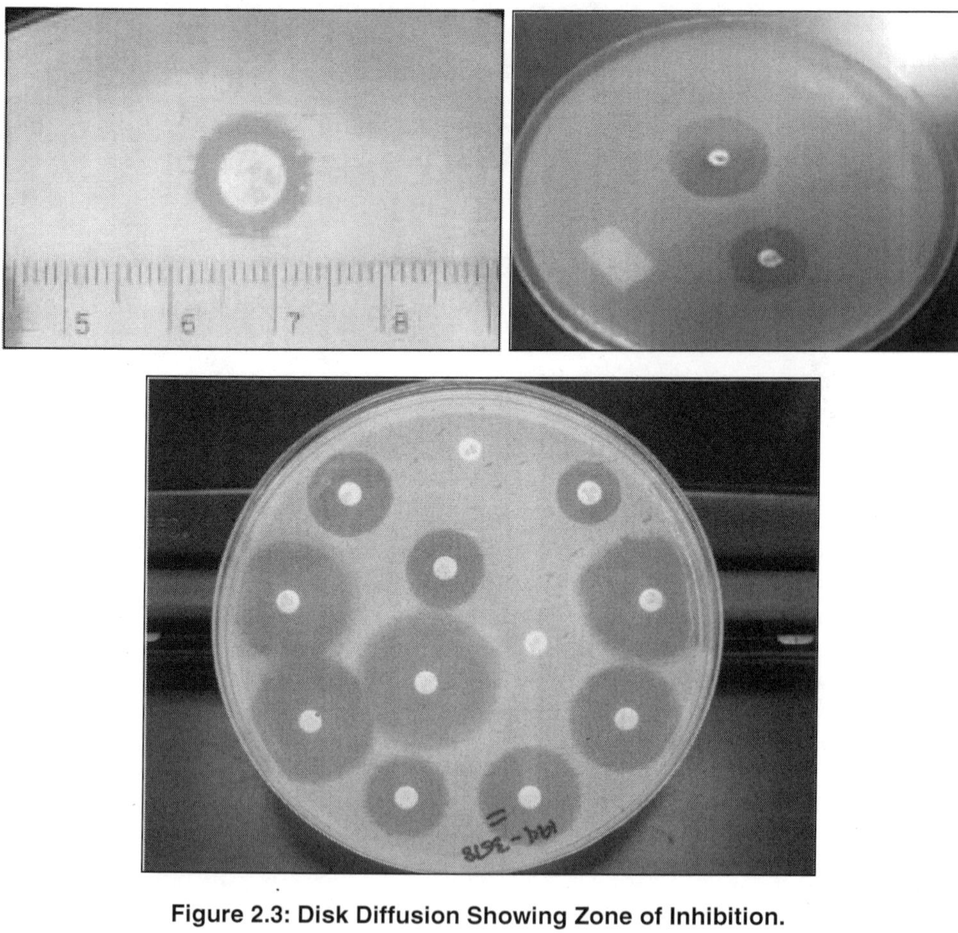

Figure 2.3: Disk Diffusion Showing Zone of Inhibition.

Quantitative Tests

Quantitative tests depend on the Minimum Inhibitory Concentration (MIC), which are recommended dor examining the microbes isolated from the food products,. MIC is the lowest concentration of antibiotic which inhibit the growth of micro-organism under specified conditions[4]. MIC values are used to estimate the susceptibilities of micro-organism towards the antibiotics and also analyze the activities of new antimicrobials. Quantitative tests include the Agar dilution method and broth dilution method.

1. Agar Dilution Method

This method is performed by applying different concentrations of antimicrobial agents on the nutrient agar plate followed by the application of a definite number of bacterial cells on the agar medium. The agar dilution method is used to examine simultaneously large number of bacterial isolates under defined conditions but it is not suitable for examining the susceptibility of the large number of antibiotics for the limited number of bacterial cells[4].

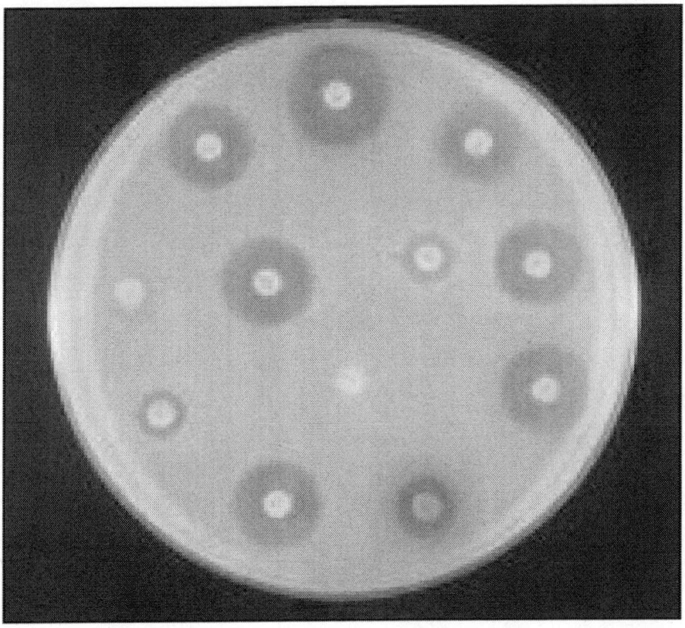

Figure 2.4: Agar Dilution Method.

Procedure

1. Prepare Mueller-Hinton Agar medium according to the manufacturer's instruction.
2. Autoclave it at 121°C,15 mins,1 bar, cool it down to 50°C.
3. Calculate the amount of antibiotic solutions needed after the cooling of the medium.

4. Label the sterile containers with the final antibiotic concentration.
5. Dispense the antibiotic solutions in the respective sterile container.
6. Add 25 ml agar into the container for each agar plate, mix well to avoid the bubbles, poured 25 ml agar into the petridish labeled with the respective concentration of the antimicrobial agent.
7. Prepare a control agar plate without any antibiotics.
8. Allow the agar plate to set.
9. Inoculate the antibiotic containing agar plates with the different concentration of antibiotics starting with the lowest concentration.
10. Incubate the agar plate in the incubator at 37°C for 16-24 hrs.
11. Count the colonies the next day.

2. Broth Dilution Method

In this method, a liquid medium is used in place of a solid agar medium with the addition of antimicrobial agents at a definite concentration. This method has an advantage over the agar dilution method as this method can be performed for testing different antimicrobial agents as well as large number of bacterial isolates. Broth dilution method can be categorized as broth macrodilution and broth microdilution method.

Broth Macrodilution Method

it is the first method which is developed for determining the MIC but now it is not much use because it is very demanding and expensive than broth microdilution method[3].

Procedure

1. In sterile test tube, prepare dilutions of antibiotic in sterile Mueller-Hinton Broth (MHB).
2. For every bacterial isolate, label the fresh sterile test tube with the antibiotic concentration to be tested. Also made control test tubes.
3. For each bacterial isolate to be tested, add 1 ml antibiotic dilution into one test tube. Add 1ml of sterile MHB into the control test tubes without antibiotic.
4. Add 1ml of bacterial suspension to the test tubes containing different dilutions of antibiotic concentration and also in the one of the control test tube (growth control).
5. Incubate the broth dilutions in the shaker incubator at 225 rpm, 37°C for 16-24 hrs.
6. After 16-24 hrs, count the colonies.

Broth Microdilution Method

In this method, 96- well microtitre plate is used instead of test tubes.

Procedure

1. 96 well microtitre plate is used, if not cover with lid, cover it with another microtiter plate.
2. Label the plate with different concentrations of antibiotic.
3. Inoculate each well containing antibiotic solution and the control growth well with the bacterial suspension.
4. Incubate the microtiter plate at 37°C.

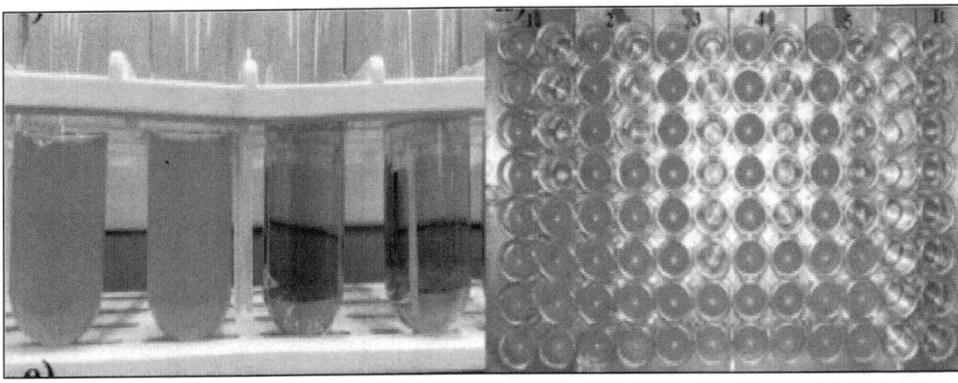

Figure 2.5: Broth Macrodilution and Microdilution Test.

3. E-Test

Epsilometer test (ETest) is a commercialized test in which plastic strips are impregnated with a gradually decreasing concentration of a specified antibiotic. MIC values are read as the point where the growth inhibition ellipse intersects the MIC scale on the strips. Bolmstrom and Eriksson develop this test in the late 1980s[5]. Cost of this test is high as a separate strip is needed for each antibiotic. It is a convenient quantitative test of antibiotic resistance of clinical isolate.

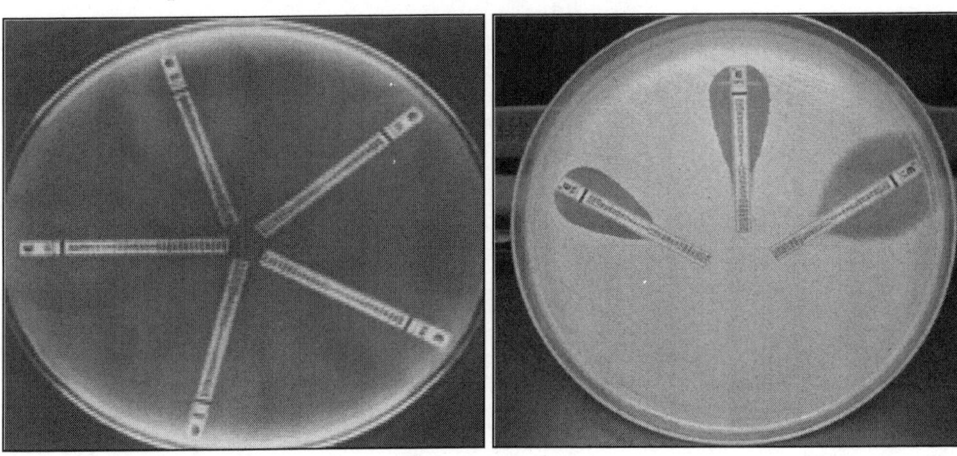

Figure 2.6: E Test.

4. Automatic Antimicrobial Susceptibility Testing Systems

Several automated commercial systems available in the laboratories for testing the antimicrobial susceptibility that provides conveniently prepared and formatted microdilution panels. One of the main advantage of this method is reduces error and lengthy preparation time.

Automatic inoculation, reading and interpretation is the main merit of most of the automated antimicrobial susceptibility testing systems. Some results can be produced within an hour and it is very convenient. One of the major drawback of this system is the cost of the system, operation and maintenance of the machine.

Some examples of these include Vitek System (bioMerieux, France), Walk-Away System (Dade International, Sacramento, Calif.), Sensititre ARIS (Trek Diagnostic Systems, East Grinstead, UK), Avantage Test System (Abbott Laboratories, Irving, Texas), Micronaut (Merlin, Bornheim-Hesel, Germany), Phoenix (BD Biosciences, Maryland) and many more.

5. Molecular Methods

Antimicrobial resistance can be detected through genotypic methods as the resistance traits are genetically encoded and many genes are responsible for antibiotic resistance. This nucleic acid based system is rapid and sensitive.

- **Polymerase chain reaction :** it is a great diagnostic tool not only for detection of microbe but also for the characterization of its resistance and virulence genotype. PCR takes 12 hr to identify the microbe and consist of 3 steps. Firstly, extraction of the genetic material of bacteria is done then, amplification of nucleic acid and lastly detection of genetic material in the agarose gel electrophoresis.

  Real-time PCR can produce results in few hours as amplification and identification of amplicons synthesis take place at the same time through different methods[6]. Several real time PCR are available commercialkt which can detect different pathogenic bacteria and their genes which are responsible for antimicrobial resistance.

- The NucliSENS EasyQ KPC platform (bioMérieux) detects genes that encode KPC carbapenemases in 2 h[7]. The Xpert Carba-Rcartridge from GeneXpert detects genes that encode KPC, NDM,VIM, IMP and OXA-48 carbapenemases in an hour are some of commercially automated available real time PCR[8].

- **DNA Hybridization:** this method is based on the principle that DNA pyrimidines hybridize with purines. Therefore, the sequence of labeled probe (specific sequence) is paired with the sequence of opened DNA of test sample because they are complementary to each other. As the hybridization occurs, probe labeled with detectable radioactive isotope, antigenic substrate or enzyme produces signals or if hybridization does not occur, it does not produce any signal.

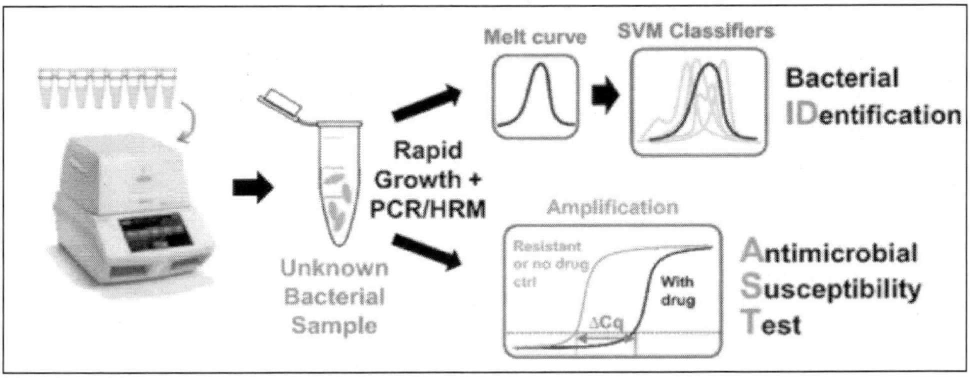

Figure 2.7: Digital-PCR High Resolution Melting Analysis (HRM) based Bacterial Identification from Mixed Bacterial Samples.

6. Mechanism-Specific Test

Antimicrobial resistance can also be detectd through tests that can directly measure the presence of the resistance mechanism of bacteria. β-lactamase is one such resistance mechanism of bacteria that can widely used against β-lactam antibiotics, which attack on penicillin binding proteins involved in bacterial cell wall synthesis. B-lactamase enzyme present in the bacteria hydrolyze the β-lactam ring which is essential for the function of antibiotic.

B-lactamase Enzyme Activated Fluorophore (β-LEAF) is one such rapid optical method for the detection of β-lactamse activity and is based on fluorophore quenching and dequenching.

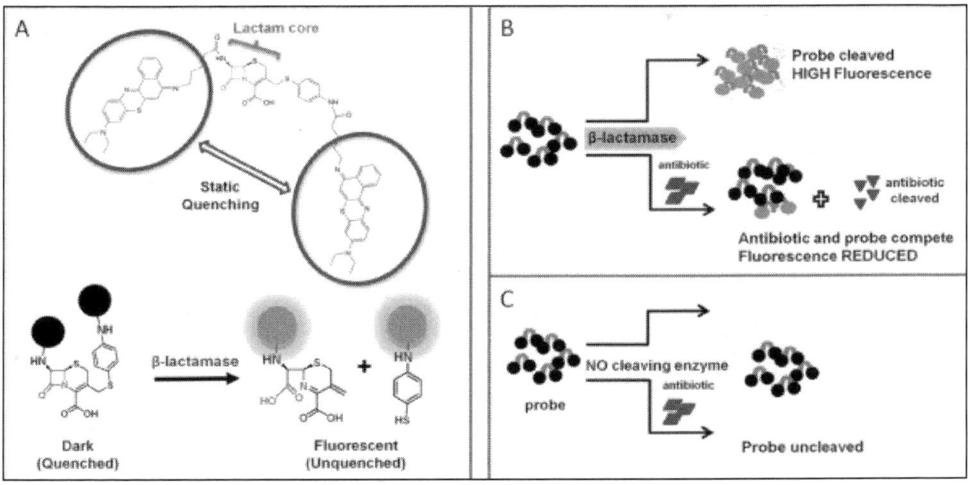

Figure 2.8: A: β-LEAF Probe made up of β-lactam Core Structure Including the Cleavable β-lactam Ring Flanked by Two Fluorophores, which undergo Static Quenching when Probe is Intact. Following cleavage β-lactamse, fluorophore moves apart and show fluoroscenes. B: Assay for β lactamase enzyme producing bacteria. C: Assay for non–β-lactamse producing bacteria.

This assay shows the use of fluorescent probes for the detection of resistance and antibiotic activity. In this assay, the structure of β-lactam ring is mimic by the prototype β-LEAF construct. This construct is made up of cephalosporin (β-lactam) core structure, with cleavable lactam ring which conjugated to two fluorophore moieties[9]. The two fluorophore moieties are in close apposition with the core structure in the ground state(quenching) (Figure 2.8A) As the time passes, β-lactamase enzyme dissociate the β-LEAF to produce two dequenched fluorophore moieties which is indicated by the increase in the fluorescence.

When both β-lactam ring and β-LEAF are present, they compete for the β-lactamase enzyme due to structural similarity. Therefore, less fluorescence is produced due to less cleavage of β-LEAF, compared to when β-LEAF is present alone (Figure 2.8C).

Conclusion

Antimicrobial resistance has become an alarming situation for the world. Despite using the measure to control the AMR around the world, it has increase tremendously due to several reasons like indiscriminate use of antibiotics, over the counter sale of antibiotics *etc.* Several measures should be taken to restrict the antimicrobial resistance. Identification and determination of AMR is one such approach to combat the antimicrobial resistance. Conventional and advanced technologies help to eliminate AMR around the world. Conventional methods are of low cost, easy to perform, no such manual power is required in operation while advanced technologies like molecular methods (PCR, DNA hybridization) are expensive, skill is required to perform, machine-based technology.

REFRENCES

1. Aminov RI.2010: A brief history of the antibiotic era: lessons learned and challenges for the future. *Front Microbiol.,* 1: 134.
2. Hoge CW., Gambel JM., and Srijan A.,1998. Trends in antibiotic resistance among diarrheal pathogens isolated in Thailand over 15 years. *Clin Infect Dis.,* **26**: 341–345.
3. Ferraro J. H. J., and Jorgensen M. J.2009. Antimicrobial Susceptibility Testing: A Review of General Principles and Contemporary Practices. *Clin. Infec. Dis.,* **7750**, 1749–1755.
4. Wiegand I., Hilpert K., and Hancock R. E. W. 2008. Agar and broth dilution methods to determine the minimal inhibitory concentration (MIC) of antimicrobial substances. *Nature Protocols,* **3**(2), 163–75.
5. Picard, J 1990. Applied Veterinary Bacteriology and Mycology: Bacteriological Techniques; University of Pretoria, Afrivip: Pretoria, South Africa.
6. March Rosselló GA, and Bratos Pérez MA. 2016. Antibiograma rápido en MicrobiologíaClínica. Enferm *Infecc Microbiol Clin.*;**34**: 61–8.3
7. Spanu T, Fiori B, d'Inzeo T, Canu G, Campoli S. and Giani T, 2012. Evaluation of the New NucliSENS EasyQ KPC test for rapid detection of Klebsiella pneumoniaecarbapenemase genes (blaKPC). *J Clin Microbiol.*;**50**: 2783–5.

8. Findlay J, Hopkins KL, Meunier D. and Woodford N. 2015. Evaluation of three commercialassays for rapid detection of genes encoding clinically relevant carbapenemasesin cultured bacteria. *J Antimicrob Chemother.*;**70:** 1338–42.

9. Munita JM., and Arias CA. 2016. Mechanisms of antibiotic resistance. *Microbiol Spectr;***4**: VMBF– 0016-2015

10. Zheng X, Sallum UW, Verma S, Athar H, Evans CL and Hasan T. 2009: Exploiting a Bacterial Drug-Resistance Mechanism: A Light-Activated Construct for the Destruction of MRSA. *Angew Chem Int Ed Engl,* **121(12)**: 2182–2185.

Chapter 4

Determination of the Minimum Inhibitory Concentration of Antibiotics

The term antibiotic was first introduced by Salmon Waksman in 1941. Antibiotics are low molecular weight microorganisms metabolites, which can have the ability or capacity to inhibit or kills microbial growth.

Alexander flaming in 1929, first time recorded the antibiotic activity. He observed the lytic effect of the mould colony (*Penicillium notatum*) on neighbouring Staphyloccocal colonies on a culture plate. Later on many antibiotics are discovered.

An antibiotic is a substance of biological, semisynthetic or synthetic origin (the last strictly on the antibacterial chemotherapeutic agent), that shows selective activity against bacteria, and is thus of potential use in the treatment of infection.

Antibiotics are antimicrobial agents produced by microorganisms that inhibit the expansion or kill other microorganisms while being harmless to the host cells. The determination of the susceptibility of pathogens to antibiotics is necessary for the selection of the most appropriate one for treating microbial infections. Antibiotics are defined as substance which kill bacteria are said to be **bactericidal**, whereas that only check their multiplication is referred to as **bacteriostatic**. However, some of the antibiotics have both the properties and act as both bacteriostatic and bactericidal, this depending upon their concentration. Which are the least concentration of antimicrobial agent that prevents microbial growth, as well as the determination of minimum bactericidal concentration (MBC), which is the least concentration of antimicrobial agent required to kill microorganisms [1].

Minimum inhibitory concentrations (MICs) are defined as the lowest concentration of an antimicrobial that will inhibit the visible growth of a microorganism after overnight incubation. MICs are employed by diagnostic laboratories mainly to verify resistance, but most often as a research tool to work out the in vitro activity of new antimicrobials, and data from such studies are wont to determine MIC breakpoints. Minimum inhibitory concentrations (MICs) are considered the 'gold standard' for determining the susceptibility of organisms to antimicrobials and are therefore wont to judge the performance of all other methods of susceptibility testing. MICs are utilized in diagnostic laboratories to verify unusual resistance, to offer a definitive answer, when a borderline result is obtained by other methods of testing. The range of antibiotic concentrations used for determining MICs is universally accepted to be in doubling dilution steps up and down from 1 mg/L as needed. The MIC is defined because of the lowest concentration of a drug which will inhibit the visible growth of an organism after overnight incubation (this period is extended for organisms such as anaerobes, which require prolonged incubation for growth). There are other definitions of MBC, and it is thus important to indicate which definition is being used.

Minimum bactericidal concentrations (MBCs) because of lowest concentration of antimicrobial that will prevent the expansion of an organism after subculture on to antibiotic-free media. MBC determinations are undertaken less frequently and their major use has been reserved for isolates from the blood of patients with endocarditis.

The optimum bactericidal concentration (OBC) or most bactericidal concentration is the concentration of antibiotic that results in the maximum proportionate kill within a given time.

The minimum serum inhibitory concentration (titre) is that reciprocal of the highest dilution (titre) of a serum sample from a patient or volunteer (dosed with an antibiotic), that prevents an increase in the number of organisms capable of reproduction within a defined period of time. It is usually expressed as the titre that prevents an increase in turbidity of a liquid culture on incubation.

The minimum serum bactericidal concentration (titre) is that reciprocal of the very best dilution (titre) of a serum sample from a patient or volunteer, that is able to reduce the number of organisms capable of reproduction as colony-forming units (cfu), usually by 99.9 per cent) (3 logarithms), within a defined period of time.

The minimum antibacterial concentration (MAC) is the concentration of an antibiotic, below the MIC as defined above, that can exert specified biological effects on bacteria.

The fractional inhibitory concentration and the fractional bactericidal concentration are mathematical expressions of the effect of the combination of antibacterial agents

An indifferent effect of a combination of antibiotics or antibiotics and inactive substances, is one that is equal to the effects of the individual substances. If one substance is more active than the other, indifference IS difficult to differentiate from an additive effect, especially when doubling dilutions of antibiotic are used.

Antagonism is present if a reduced effect of a mixture of antibiotics is observed as compared with the effect of the foremost individual substance.

Traditional antibiotic dosage adjustments target predetermined serum concentrations, whereas a number of in vitro studies and updated clinical trials establish that bacteria vary in their susceptibility. Dual individualization, which considers the variance in both antibiotic pharmacokinetics and bacteria susceptibility, has been employed to explain different rates of bacterial eradication in reference to varying serum concentrations.

Procedure

The agar dilution technique is used to measure qualitatively the in vitro activity of an antimicrobial agent against the test bacteria. In this method, graded amounts of antibiotics are incorporated in agar plates and inoculated in spots with the organisms under study. If the organism under study is susceptible to the incorporated antibiotic, no bacterial growth is expected in agar plates with higher amounts of the drugs. Bacterial growth is observed as the antibiotic concentration in the agar plate diminishes. Inhibition of growth at the minimum or lowest concentration of antibiotic is regarded as the end point.

The minimal inhibitory concentration (MIC) test is performed using Mueller-Hinton Agar (MHA), which is the best medium for routine susceptibility tests because it has good reproducibility, low in sulfonamide, trimethoprim, and tetracycline inhibitors, and gives satisfactory growth of most bacterial pathogens.

The inoculum is prepared using a suitable broth such as heart infusion broth (HIB). This medium is prepared according to the manufacturer's instructions, dispensed in tubes at 3 ml and sterilized. Sterile 0.9 per cent salt solution may also be used. Media supplemented with 1-2 per cent sodium chloride (NaCl) if intended for marine species [2].

Preparation of Antimicrobial Agent Stock Solution

1. Remove the antimicrobial agent from the freezer, and warm to room temperature before opening to avoid condensation of water.
2. Weigh the appropriate amount of the powdered antimicrobial agent.
3. Dissolve the antimicrobial agent powder in solvent to make a concentration of 1,000 µg/ml.

   NOTE: Stock Solutions

   a. At least 1,000 µg/ml or 10 times the highest concentration to be tested is to be prepared as an antimicrobial agent stock solution. Some antimicrobial agents are of limited solubility.

      Therefore, lower concentration may be required. However, in all cases, drug manufacturers provide directions for determining solubility.

   b. Some drugs must be dissolved in solvents other than water. In such cases, it is necessary to:

1) Use only enough solvent to dissolve the antimicrobial agent powder;

2) Dilute to the final stock concentration with distilled water.

3) Prepare appropriate volumes of distilled water, the desired volume for serial dilution.

4. Dispense the stock solution into sterile diluent using a two-fold dilution technique.

   NOTE: As an example, a range of 0.012-100 µg/ml two-fold dilutions may be used as test concentrations for different antibiotics. For Sulfadimethoxine and Sulfadiazine, 400 µg/ml may be used as the highest test concentration

4. Set aside.

Preparation of Antimicrobial Agar Plates

1. Label each empty sterile plate in order to identify the antimicrobial agent and their concentrations.

   Example: 0. 024 OTC means 0.024 µg/ml of oxytetracycline
2. Place the label on the upper portion of the bottom side of the petri dish to ensure that the plate is inserted at the correct point of the basal stand A of the multiple inoculating apparatus.
3. Draw a scheme to locate each bacterial strain in a well on a reference paper that will be used to read the results.
4. Prepare MHA following manufacturer's direction and supplement with 1-2 per cent NaCl, if intended for marine organisms. Keep in a water bath at 48-50°C until use.
5. Pipette 1 ml of appropriate dilutions of the test antimicrobial agent
6. Pipette 9 ml of MHA (keep warm at 48- 50°C), add into the plate with the appropriate dilution of the test antimicrobial agent and mix thoroughly.
7. Allow the agar to solidify at room temperature and use the plates immediately after the agar surface has dried completely. If necessary, dry the surface of the agar in a laminar flow chamber under UV light, but avoid excessive drying [3].

Control Agar Plates/Drug Free Agar Plates

Prepare control agar plates by pipetting 10 ml of MHA into a sterile petri dish. Do not add any antimicrobial agent. There should at least be 2 control plates [2].

Preparation

1. From a pure 18-24 hour bacterial culture get 4- 5 isolated colonies (to minimize the risk of picking bacteria that have lost their resistance) and subculture to a tube with 3 ml HIB containing 0.3 per cent yeast extract and 2 per cent NaCl.

2. Shake vigorously in a water bath at 30°C until it achieves or exceeds the turbidity of 0.5 MacFarland standard (prepared by adding 0.5 ml of 0.048 M $BaCl_2$ to 99.5 ml of 0.36 NH_2SO_4; commercially available). The inoculums may also be standardized based on optical density [OD625 of 0.08-0.1 (1 cm light path)] using a spectrophotometer. This is usually achieved after 18-24 hours.
3. Dilute the standardized inoculum 1:10 in sterile saline solution to obtain the desired concentration of 10^6 cfu/ml.
4. Pipette 0.1 ml of the 10^6 cfu/ml inoculum and transfer to a well, of a multi-dispenser containing 0.9 ml of HIB with 0.3 per cent yeast extract. In the absence of a multi-dispenser (photo at right), sterile test tubes of the same size may be used to hold the diluted standardized inoculum.
5. Store at room temperature for not more than 2 hours before testing.

Inoculation Volume

Inoculate plates with 1-3 µl of the inoculum if automatic multi-dispenser is used and 10 µl if done manually. Inoculated volume should be uniform for good results.

Inoculation Sequence

1. When using automatic multiple inoculating apparatus, drug free or control plate should be inoculated first, followed by the plate with the lowest antimicrobial concentration. Inoculate a second control agar plate last to ensure that there is no contamination or antimicrobial agent carry-over during the inoculation.
2 When inoculating manually, it is only important to include a drug free or control plate at the beginning of the inoculation series.

Inoculation

1. Place a completely dried agar plate on the basal stand A of the multiple inoculating apparatus. Insert the plate on the basal stand A of the multiple inoculating apparatus in such a way that the label on the plate is facing the front direction.
2. Place the multiple well tray of the multidispenser, which contain 1 ml of inocula, onto the basal stand B to ensure that the marking on the tray is arranged at the front direction.
3. Set the tray to ensure that each inoculators stick will properly dip into the inoculum and carry a uniform volume of each test bacteria.
4. Set the apparatus to ensure that the surface of each multiple inoculators stick will properly touch the surface of the medium in the agar plate.
5. Inoculate the bacterial suspensions onto the surface of the agar plate.

Incubation

1. Let the inoculated agar plates remain at room temperature until the moisture in the inoculum spot is absorbed by the agar or until all spots are dry.
2. Incubate the plates in an inverted position at 30°C for 18-24 hours.

Reading of MIC Value

1. Lay the agar plates on a non-reflecting dark surface and observe bacterial growth with the naked eye. Place the inoculated plate on or beside the reference paper to identify the spot or position of each tested bacteria.
2. Check bacterial growth on the 2 control plates, disregard the results if no growth is observed in some control strains. The test should be repeated.
3. Read and record the MIC at the lowest concentration of antimicrobial agent that completely inhibits the growth of the organism as detected by the naked eye.
4. The MIC is the lowest concentration of antimicrobial agent that completely inhibits colony formation.
5. Disregard a single colony or a faint haze caused by the inoculum.
6. Repeat the test if two or more colonies persist in concentrations of the agent beyond an obvious end point; that is, if there is no growth at lower concentration but there is growth at higher concentrations.
7. When reporting the MIC values of antimicrobial agents that will prevent the growth of bacterial strains, include important information such as the locality and date the samples were isolated or collected.

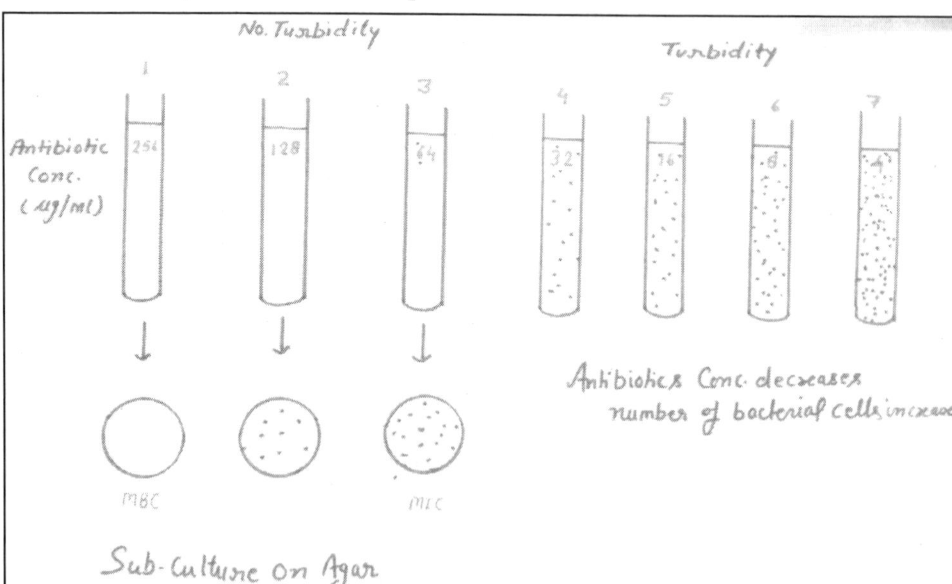

Figure 4.1: Dilution Method for MIC and MBC.

8. Evaluate the MIC range of each antimicrobial agent.
9. Compare the MIC breakpoint of the test isolates with those in the chart
10. Report result as Resistant (R), Intermediate (I) or Susceptible (S).

    Example: Antibiotic: oxytetracycline MIC breakpoint: 0.2 µg/ml Interpretation: susceptible.

How to determine the Minimum Inhibitory Concentration (MIC) and Minimum Bactericidal Concentration (MBC)

The MIC of an antibacterial agent for a specific bacterium can be determined invitro. MIC is that the lowest concentration of your drug that inhibits bacterial growth so you'll haven't any turbidity in your culture media but MBC is that the lowest concentration that kills bacteria. Then the lowest concentration of your drug that inhibits bacterial growth are going to be considered as MBC [4].

REFERENCES

1. Jennifer M. Andrews, Determination of minimum inhibitory concentrations, *Journal of Antimicrobial Chemotherapy*, Volume 49, Issue 6, June 2002, Page 1049, https: //doi.org/10.1093/jac/dkf083
2. Wiegand, I., Hilpert, K. and Hancock, R. Agar and broth dilution methods to determine the minimal inhibitory concentration (MIC) of antimicrobial substances. Nat Protoc **3**, 163–175 (2008). https: //doi.org/10.1038/nprot.2007.521
3. Ruangpan, L. (2004). Minimal inhibitory concentration (MIC) test and determination of antimicrobial resistant bacteria. In Laboratory manual of standardized methods for antimicrobial sensitivity tests for bacteria isolated from aquatic animals and environment (pp.31-55). http: //hdl.handle.net/10862/1637
4. Parvekar P, Palaskar J, Metgud S, Maria R, Dutta S. The minimum inhibitory concentration (MIC) and minimum bactericidal concentration (MBC) of silver nanoparticles against Staphylococcus aureus. *Biomater Investig Dent*. 2020;7(1): 105-109. Published 2020 Jul 23. doi: 10.1080/26415275.2020.1796674

Chapter 5

Pharmacokinetic Study Design

Introduction

The four key physiological processes that govern the time course of drug fate in (absorption), through (distribution) and out (metabolism and elimination) of the body the so called *ADME processes*. Pharmacokinetics, the study of the time course of drug concentrations in the body, provides a means of quantitating ADME parameters[1]. The study of pharmacokinetics is essential in therapeutics because it determines the route of administration, dose and onset of action time of peak effect, duration of action and frequency of drug administration[2].

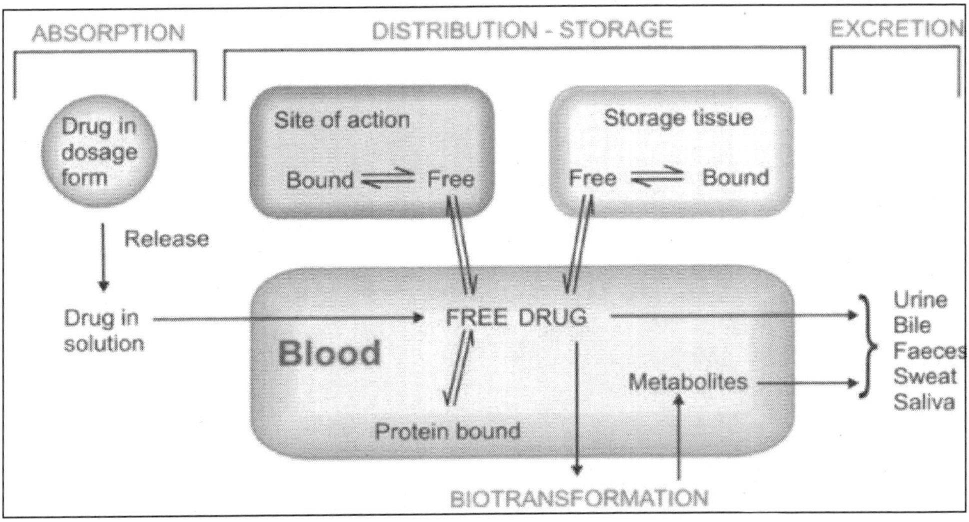

Figure 5.1: Schematic Depiction of Pharmacokinetic Processes.

Drugs are administered into the body with the aim of producing their desired effect on the target organs. Once a drug is administered at an appropriate site, it must be absorbed effectively into the blood stream, distributed efficiently to the site of action and subsequently metabolized and eliminated from the body[3]. All pharmacokinetic processes involve movement of drug across biological membranes.

Drug molecules must pass through several physiological barriers before reaching the vascular system. Biological membranes are selective molecular barriers to the body environment, which segregate organ function, separate cells from one another, and compartmentalize intracellular events. Drug transport processes have been broadly divided into two groups; Simple transport (Diffusion and Filtration) and specialized transport (Active and facilitated transport and pinocytosis).

Absorption

Absorption is the movement of an unchanged drugs from the site of administration into the blood. Except for the intravenous route, absorption is the pre-requisite for all systemic routes because the drug exerts its pharmacological action only it comes into blood stream. Both rate and extent of drug absorption are important as they determine the duration and intensity of drug action and the factors affecting the rate and extent of drug absorption are; physiochemical properties of the drug (lipid solubility, *pKa* and molecular size of the drug), nature and type of dosage form (Solutions>emulsions>suspensions>capsules>tablets>sustained release products), concentration and volume of drug (High concentration and the large volume of drug develop high concentration gradient, a pre-requisite for passive diffusion), blood flow to the site of administration (better perfusion enhances absorption), area of absorbing site (larger surface area better absorption *e.g.* Intestine>stomach) and route of drug administration *i.e.*, I/P>I/M>S/C>oral[4,7].

Distribution

It is a process by which drug reversibly leaves the blood stream and enters the extravascular fluid and tissues for metabolism and excretion.

Biotransformation

Metabolism or biotransformation is the process of conversion of lipid soluble and non-polar compounds to water-soluble and polar compounds to facilitate excretion. It is a necessary biological process that limits pharmacological action and the life of a drug in the body. The metabolites of the drug may have the same, or different, pharmacological action as the parent drug, even sometimes cause toxic side effects. Excretion is the irreversible drug removal process from the body and commonly occurs via the kidney or biliary tract. This transformation occurs inside the body hence termed specifically as biotransformation.

It causes pharmacological inactivation, which is a conversion of an active to inactive metabolites (phenytoin to *p*-hydroxyphenytoin), toxicological activation *i.e.*, conversion of an active to more active metabolites (codeine to morphine), pharmacological activation which means conversion of pro-drug to active metabolites (phenacitin to paracetamol).

Pathways of Biotransformation

Phase I (Non-conjugative or synthetic pathway): Oxidation, reduction and hydrolysis of drugs catalyzed by microsomal (aldehyde dehydrogenase *etc.*) and non microsomal enzymes (glucuronide transferase).

Excretion

It is the process of elimination of drugs or their metabolites from the body. It is an important process of termination of pharmacological effect of the drug.

Plasma Drug Concentration-Time Profile

Pharmacokinetic principles relate specifically to the variations in drug concentration as a result of pharmacokinetic processes (ADME). The speed of onset, intensity and duration of a pharmacological effect depends on the concentration of the drug at the site of action. As it is difficult to collect tissue samples, the time course of drug concentration is approximated by measuring drug concentrations in plasma. However, concentration of the drug can be measured in the blood or plasma, saliva, urine, and other fluids. The plasma drug-concentration curve is obtained by measuring the drug concentration in plasma taken at different time intervals after drug administration and then plotting the concentrations of drug at Y-axis versus the corresponding time at X-axis (Figuire 5.2).

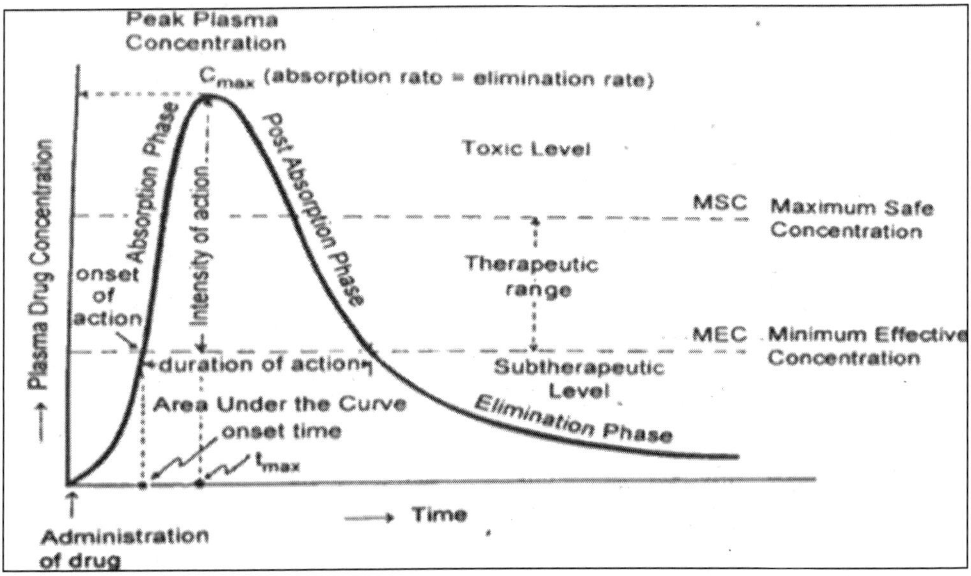

Figure 5.2: Plasma Drug-Concentration Time Curve after Single Oral Dose.

When a drug is administered by oral or extravascular route, it slowly enters systemic circulation plasma drug concentration gradually rises to maximum level. As the drug is being absorbed into the blood, it is distributed to the tissues, metabolized and simultaneously eliminated from the body. The ascending portion of the curve to left of the peak represents the absorption phase (*Ka*) because in this phase, the rate of absorption is always greater than the rate of distribution and elimination. The descending section of the curve to right represents the elimination phase (β) because rate of elimination exceeds the rate of absorption.

a. Minimum Effective Concentration (MEC): Minimum concentration of a drug in plasma required to produce the desirable pharmacological response. In case of antimicrobial drugs, the term Minimum Inhibitory Concentration (MIC) is used.
b. Maximum Safe Concentration (MSC) or Minimum Toxic Concentration (MTC): Concentration of drug in plasma above which toxic effects of the drug are produced.
c. Maximum Plasma concentration or Peak Plasma Concentration (C_{max}): The highest concentration of drug in plasma. It is the point of time when absorption rate equals elimination rate ($\mu g.ml^{-1}$).
d. Area under Curve (AUC): Total integrated area under the plasma drug-concentration time curve ($\mu g.ml^{-1}.h$).
e. Peak Effect: Maximum pharmacological effect produced by the drug.
f. Time of Maximum Concentration (t_{max}): Time required for a drug to reach maximum concentration (h).
g. The onset of Action: Beginning of pharmacological effect produced by a drug.
h. Duration of Action: Time period for which pharmacological effect is produced by a drug.

Orders of Pharmacokinetic Processes or Kinetics

It is the manner in which the concentration of a drug influences the rate of a pharmacokinetic process.

a. Zero Order Kinetics or Constant Rate Constant: Pharmacokinetic process whose rate is independent of the drug concentration. The rate remains constant and cannot be increased further by increasing the concentration of drug. A fixed amount of drug is processed per unit time. Half life is not constant and is proportional to the concentration of drug. *e.g.* constant rate I/V infusion.
b. First Order kinetics or linear Kinetics: Rate is directly proportional to the concentration of the drug *i.e.*, greater the concentration faster the process. Fixed fraction of drug is processed per unit time so half life is constant and is independent of concentration of drug. Most drugs follow linear kinetics.

Models of Pharmacokinetics

Simplifications of body processes are necessary to predict a drug's behavior in the body. One way to make these simplifications is to apply mathematical principles to the various processes. Three types of models are used; Compartmental models, non-compartment models and physiological models[5].

a. Compartment Model

The most commonly employed approach to the pharmacokinetic characterization of the drug is to represent the body as a system of compartments, even though these compartments do not exist anatomically and physiologically and to assume that the rate of transfer between compartments and the rate of elimination from compartments follow first-order kinetics.

a. One Compartment Model

The body is considered to be a single, kinetically homogenous unit. This model is used to describe plasma levels following a single dose of drug (Figure 5.3).

I/V Bolus Administration

The drug concentration time curve is obtained as a straight line on semi-logarithmic papers showing mono-phasic exponential decline due to elimination of the drug from the body. The distribution phase is neglected in calculations because distribution is very rapid. The extrapolated zero-time intercept of linear elimination phase gives the coefficient B and the elimination rate constant is given by β. The value of B is an estimate of zero-time concentration of drug in plasma represented by C^0 or Cp^0 (Fig. 4).

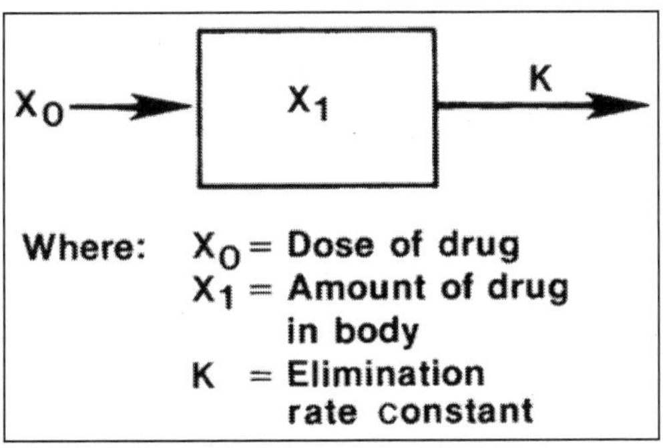

Figure 5.3: One Compartment Open Model.

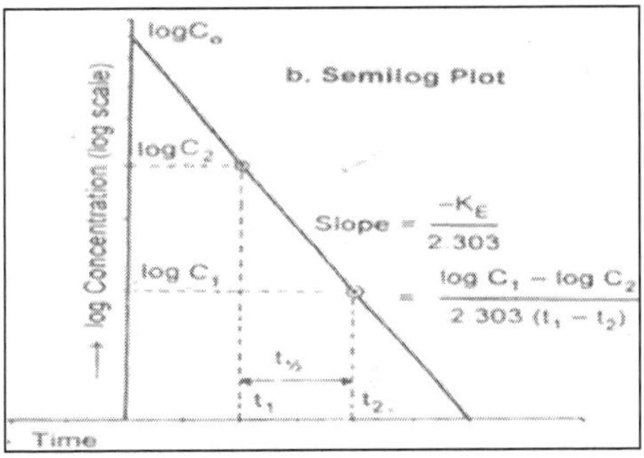

Figure 5.4: Semi-logarithmic Graph Depicting Plasma Drug Concentration Time Profile after Single I/V Administration.

Extravascular administration: Absorption is the pre-requisite for drugs given by I/M, S/C *etc.* The rate of change in drug concentration is given by two exponents-absorption constant (Ka) and (β) elimination constant (Figures 5.5 and 5.6).

ii. Two Compartment Model

The body is assumed to be composed of two compartments *viz* central (Compartment I) and peripheral compartment (Compartment II). The Central consists of blood and highly perfused organs (Liver, kidney, lungs *etc.*) and the peripheral consists of less perfused organs (skin and bones *etc.*). Drug transfer from central to peripheral compartment follow the first order kinetics and is defined by

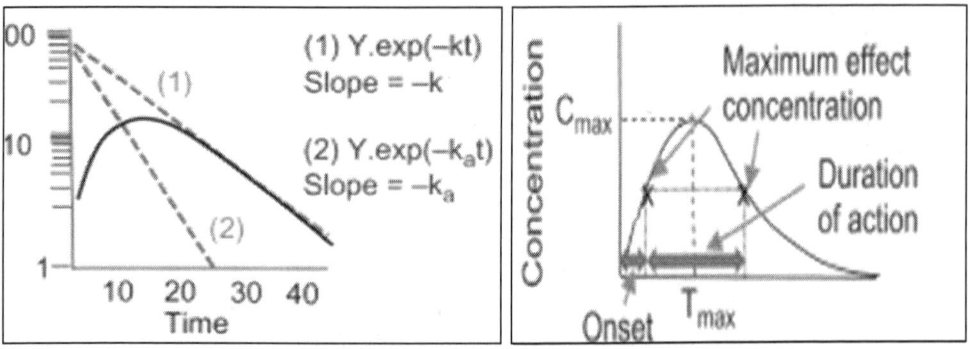

Figure 5.5 and 5.6: Semi-logarithmic Graph Depicting Plasma Drug Concentration Time Profile after Single Extra-vascular Administration of Drug.

rate constant denoted by 'k'. The subscript refers to the direction of drug movement *i.e.,* k_{12} (From central to peripheral) and vice-versa for k_{21} (Figure 5.7).

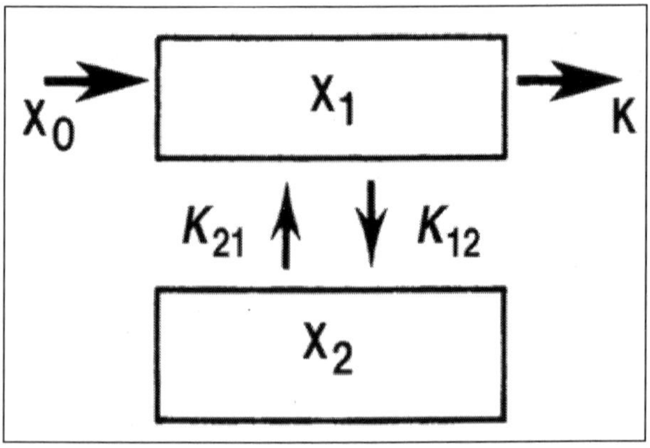

Figure 5.7: Two Compartment Open Model

Intravenous bolus administration: Plasma drug concentration decline is bi-exponential *i.e.,* decline rapidly in the first phase followed by a slow terminal decline when plasma drug-concentration time curve is plotted on the semi-logarithmic graph. The initial relatively non-linear steep decline in drug concentration is attributed to distribution of drug from central to peripheral compartment and terminal shallow decline to the elimination of drug from the central compartment. The linear terminal portion of the curve is called elimination phase (Figure 5.8). By extrapolation of the linear portion blood concentration at time 0 are calculated (C^0 or Cp^0).

When the bi-exponential curve is resolved into components by the method of residuals (feathering technique), then the distribution phase can be obtained as linear curve known as distribution phase denoted by 'A' and elimination phase by 'B'. The distribution rate constant is denoted by 'α' and 'β' is elimination rate constant. The coefficients (A and B) and rate constants (α and β) are calculated from the experimental data by least square regression analysis (Figure 5.8).

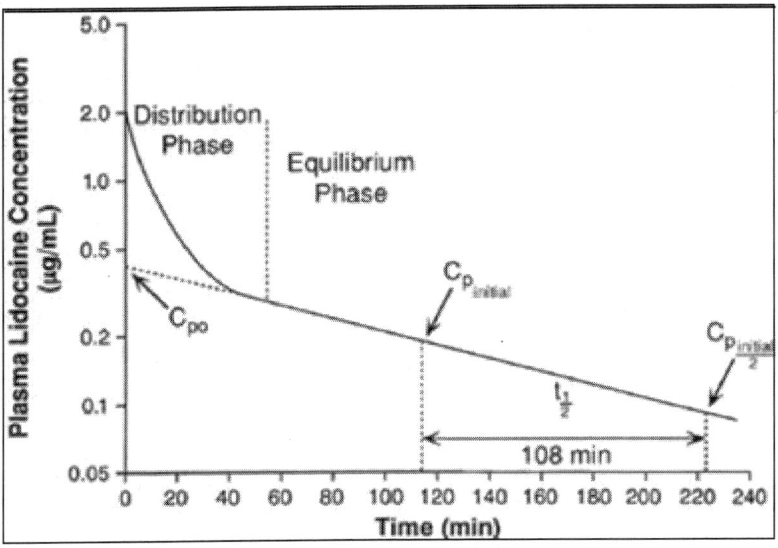

Figure 5.8: Semi-logarithmic Graph Depicting Plasma Drug Concentration Time Profile after Single I/V Administration.

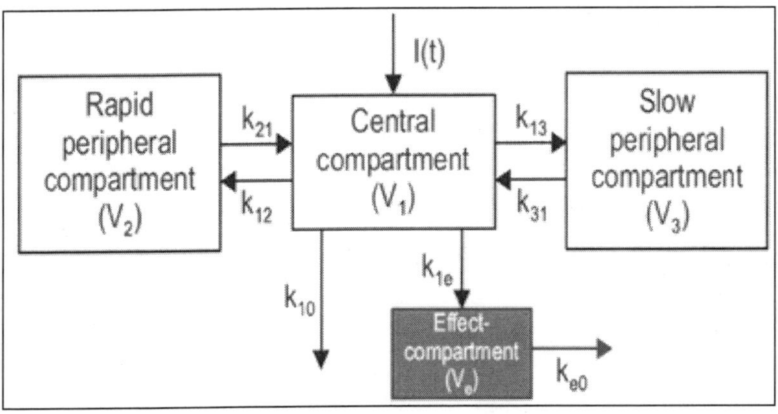

Figure 5.9: Three Compartment Open Model.

b. Non-Compartmental Model

Non-compartmental analysis is another approach to study the time course of drug in the body. Basically there are two forms of the non-compartmental model: the single accessible pool model and the two accessible pool models. The non-compartmental approach does not require any specific compartmental model for the system to analyze the pharmacokinetic data also it can be applied to any pharmacokinetic data and does not require a detailed description of drug disposition. It considers the time course of drug concentration in plasma as a statistical distribution curve and derives pharmacokinetic parameters by simple algebraic equations. The disadvantage of this method is that it often deals with averages and provides limited information regarding plasma drug-concentration time profile. This approach is a primary pharmacokinetic data analysis method for pharmaceutical industries because of its versatility[3, 5].

Design of Dosage Regimen

Dosage regimen is the manner in which a drug is administered. For some drugs single dose may provide effective treatment (anaethetics, antiemetics *etc.*). In such cases, there is no chance of drug accumulation and a constant therapeutic plasma concentration is no required. However, for many drugs like antimicrobials, multidoses of the drug at appropriate intervals over a period of time are required for successful therapy. A dosage regimen is composed of two important variables: Dose size (the magnitude of each dose and dosing interval (the frequency with which the dose is repeated).

Dose

Dose or dose size is a quantitative term estimating the amount of drug, which should be administered to produce a particular biological response *i.e.* to achieve a specified target plasma concentration of drug. The size of the dose should be selected that it produces the peak plasma concentration (C_{max}) within the limits of the therapeutic range (between minimum effective concentration and maximum safe concentration).

Dosing Interval

The dosing interval is the time interval between doses. It ensures maintenance of plasma concentration of a drug within the therapeutic range for the entire duration of therapy.

Steady-state Concentration (C_{ss})

It is the time during which the concentration remains consistent when the drug is given repeatedly or continuously (I/V infusion). The time to reach steady state is a function of elimination half life ($t_{½}$) and is achieved when the rate of drug entering into the systemic circulation equals the rate of elimination.

Multiple Dosing

When a drug is administered in a fixed dose at fixed intervals, the plasma concentration rises exponentially to a plateau or steady state with a half time of increase that is equal to the elimination half-life of the drug.

Collection of Sample after Drug Administration

For the entire concentration, 5 to 7 time sampling is required. In early distribution phase at least two times within 15 min after injection is recommended and in terminal phase at least three to five times is required for reliable estimation of the terminal half-life of a drug. In general, not more than 10 per cent of the total blood volume in the body of small animals can be drawn. It is acceptable weekly in the case of small laboratory animals.

Collection of urine in laboratory animals over an extended period of time (usually up to 24 hr) can also provide useful pharmacokinetic information such as renal clearance and metabolic profiles of a drug.

Following parameters are calculated in Pharmacokinetics[8]:

B - The overall elimination rate constant and expressed as h^{-1}.β = 2.303 m; where, 'm' is the slope and calculated by the least square regression method.

B - Zero time intercept of the least square regression line of the elimination (β) phase and represents the expected zero time plasma concentration ($\mu g.ml^{-1}$) of the drug.

A - Distribution rate constant and expressed as h^{-1}.

α = 2.303 m;

Where the slope 'm' is calculated by the feathering technique.

A - Zero time intercept of the least square regression line of the distribution phase (α) and expressed as $\mu g.ml^{-1}$.

Ka - The absorption rate constant and expressed as h^{-1}.

Ka = 2.303 m;Where the slope 'm' is calculated by feathering technique.

A - Zero time intercept of the least square regression line of the absorption phase (Ka) and expressed as $\mu g.ml^{-1}$.

$t_{1/2}\beta$ - Elimination half-life, expressed in h.

$$\text{Half} - \text{life}\left(t_{1/2}\right) = 0.\frac{693}{\text{Rate constant}}$$

Cp^0 - The theoretical expected plasma drug concentration ($\mu g.ml^{-1}$) at zero time following a single intravenous administration.

AUC - Total area under the plasma drug concentration time curve and expressed as $\mu g.ml^{-1}.h$.

$$AUC = \left(\frac{A}{\alpha} + \frac{B}{\beta}\right)$$ (Two compartment)

$$AUC = \frac{B}{\beta} - \frac{A'}{Ka}$$ (Extravascular route one compartment)

MRT - Mean residence time and expressed in h.

$$MRT = \frac{AUMC}{AUC}$$

K_{el} - The elimination rate constant of the drug from the central compartment and is expressed as h^{-1}.

$$K_{el} = \frac{Cp^0}{AUC}$$

K_{12} - The elimination rate constant of the drug from the central compartment and is expressed as h^{-1}.

$K_{12} = \alpha+\beta-K_{21}-K_{el}$

K_{21} - The rate constant of the transfer of drug from peripheral compartment to central compartment and expressed in h^{-1}.

$$K_{21} = \frac{A\beta + \alpha B}{Cp^{\circ}}$$

C_{max} - Observed peak plasma concentration of the drug and expressed as $\mu g.ml^{-1}$.

t_{max} - Observed time at which peak plasma concentration is achieved.

V_c - Apparent volume of the central compartment and expressed as $L.Kg^{-1}$.

$$V_c = \frac{Dose}{Cp^{\circ}} \quad a$$

Vd - Apparent volume of the distribution of drug and expressed as $L.Kg^{-1}$

Vd_B - Apparent volume of distribution based on the zero time plasma drug concentration intercept of the least square regression line of elimination phase by neglecting the distribution or absorption phase(s) of drug disposition and expressed as $L.Kg^{-1}$.

Vd_{area} - Apparent volume of distribution of drug based on total area under the plasma drug concentration versus time curve and expressed as $L.Kg^{-1}$.

$$Vd_{area} = \frac{Dose}{\beta \times AUC} \text{ (Intravascular route)}$$

$$Vd_{area} = \left(\frac{Dose}{\beta \times AUC}\right) \times F \text{ (Extravascular route)}$$

Vd_{ss} - Steady state volume of distribution of the drug and expressed as $L.kg^{-1}$.

$$Vd_{SS} = \frac{Dose \times AUMC}{AUC^2}$$

Cl_B - Total body clearance of the drug and expressed as $L.kg.^{-1}h^{-1}$.

$Cl_B = V_C \times K_{el}$ (Intravenous route)

$Cl_B = Vd_{(area)} \times \beta$ (Intramuscular route)

C_{max}/MIC - Ratio of the observed peak plasma concentration and minimum inhibitory concentration (MIC) of the drug.

AUIC - Area under the inhibitory plasma drug concentration time curve.

$$AUIC = \frac{AUC_{(route)}}{MIC}$$

F - Bioavailability of the drug after extravascular administration and expressed in per cent.

$$F = \frac{AUC_{(extravascular)}}{AUC_{i.v}} \times 100$$

REFERENCES

1. Riviere, J. E. and Papich, M. G. (2009). Absorption, Distribution, Metabolism and Elimination. In: *Veterinary Pharmacology and Therapeutics*, 9th ed., Riviere, J. E., Papich, M. G. and Adams, H. R. (Eds.), Wiley Blackwell, 2121 State Avenue, Ames, Iowa 50014-8300, USA. pp: 2046-2103.

2. Durairaj, C. (2016). Ocular Pharmacokinetics. In: Handbook of Experimental Pharmacology Springer International Publishing Switzerland 2016 S.M. Whitcup, D.T. Azar (eds.), Pharmacologic Therapy of Ocular Disease, 242, DOI 10.1007/164_2016_32.

3. Sandhu, H.S. (2018). Principles and Basic Concepts of Pharmacokinetics. In: *Essentials of Veterinary Pharmacology and Therapeutics*. 2nd Edn India. ISBN 978-93-272-2824-3.

4. Lin, L. and Wong, H. (2017). Predicting Oral Drug Absorption: Mini Review on Physiologically-Based Pharmacokinetic Models. *Pharmaceutics*, **9**(4): 1-14.

5. Foster, D.M. (2007). Noncompartmental versus Compartmental Approaches to Pharmacokinetic Analysis. In: Principles of Clinical Pharmacology. 2nd Edn, Arthur J. Atkinson, Darrell R. Abernethy, Charles E. Daniels, Robert L. Dedrick, Sanford P. Markey, (Second Edition), Academic Press, pp 89-105, ISBN 9780123694171.

6. Gibaldi, M. and Perrier, D. (2007). Pharmacokinetics. 2nd edn., Marcel Deccar lnc., New York (USA).

7. Alagga AA, Gupta V. Drug Absorption. (2020). In: StatPearls. Treasure Island (FL): StatPearls Publishing. Available from: https: //www.ncbi.nlm.nih.gov/books/NBK557405.

8. Baggot, J. D. (2001). The Physiological Basis of Veterinary Clinical Pharmacology, Blackwell Science Ltd., UK. ISBN 0-632-05744-0.

Chapter 6

Tissue Organ Bath System

Isolated tissue and organ preparations have been in use for over one hundred years, providing researchers with suitable biological models. That exists without the systemic influences of the intact animal under controlled a environment. The recent development of transgenic animal models and pharmacological drugs testing has extended the scope of isolated tissue organ bath system.

Basic Principles

To create a useful experimental isolated tissue and organ preparation one must construct a system that permits the optimal performance of the tissue in a controlled environment. Changes in tissue function can be recorded by instrument. The researcher firstly determines (a) the specific aims and hypotheses of the research (b) the animal species and tissue type that would be suitable research models (c) the kinds of experimental responses. (d) the instruments, methods, and statistical analysis required to measure and analyze these results.

The organ bath is an instrument commonly used in vitro dose response experiments and to investigate the physiology and pharmacology of in vitro tissue preparations. In an organ bath an isolated piece of tissue can be kept alive for many hours, allowing for detailed investigations into how substances added to the tissue influence functional responses in a temperature controlled environment. The tissue in the organ bath is typically oxygenated with carbogen (a mixture of 95 per cent oxygen and 5 per cent carbon dioxide) and kept in a solution such as Tyrode's solution or lactated Ringer's solution. Historically, they have also been called gut baths.

Initially, organ baths were developed to study classical excitable tissue such as axons and muscles, but they have been adapted to study epithelia and all manner of intercellular communication. The organ bath is most commonly used to study the actions of drugs in vitro to characterize their properties as agonists or antagonists.

Although organ bath approaches can be applied to a variety of mammalian and non-mammalian tissues and organs, the most widely used approach utilizes muscle contraction as the functional measure. Studies investigating neuronal function can measure the consequence of neuronal input and transmitter release through muscle contraction or by directly recording electrical activity. Part of smooth muscles from different body tissues like ileum,[2] colon,[3] vas deferens,[4] trachea,[5] bladder,[6] corpus cavernosum,[7] and blood vessels such as aortic rings. The contraction of smooth muscle tissues can be readily measured with a myograph; this type of physiological response is more readily quantifiable than that of other tissues. Organ baths were originally developed to study the effects of agonists and antagonists on excitable tissues, such as nervous tissue and muscle though they have been adapted to study tissues such as epithelium.[8] Typical tissues and receptors studied with organ bath preparations include nicotinic, muscarinic and histamine receptors in the ileum or beta adrenoceptors in the bladder.[8] Tissues are typically taken from rodents, such as guinea pigs, mice and rats.

For studying the effects of drugs on receptors in drug discovery and combinatorial chemistry, novel techniques such as high throughput screening, ultra high throughput screening, and high content screening, pharmacogenomics, proteomics and array technology have largely superseded the use of organ baths.[9] These techniques can allow more receptor specificity than organ bath preparations, as a single tissue sample can express many different receptor types.

The use of organ bath preparations for the measurement of physiological tissue responses to drug concentrations allows the generation of dose response curves. This in turn allows the quantification of a drug's pharmacological profile in the tissue in question, such as the calculation of the drug's EC50, IC50, and Hill coefficient.

In pharmacological studies, a range of concentrations of the drug of interest are tested alone or in combination with another drug treatment and the data are analyzed to generate concentration-response curves. When planning an experiment using an organ bath, a number of key considerations must be addressed:

1. Choice of tissue, physiological salt solution and experimental equipment.
2. Drugs and the concentration range to use.
3. Specific experimental objective, *e.g.*, agonist potency, antagonist affinity, receptor profile of the tissue, pharmacological profile of a novel compound, bioassay. For example:
    a) An experiment to compare the agonist potency of different drugs acting at muscarinic acetylcholine receptors would investigate a range of concentrations in a tissue such as the isolated ileum preparation.
    b) An experiment to investigate the function of an ion channel associated with an action potential would use a tissue such as the isolated frog sciatic nerve.

Parts of a Typical Organ Bath System

Various parts of a typical organ bath system are presented in the Figure 6.1.

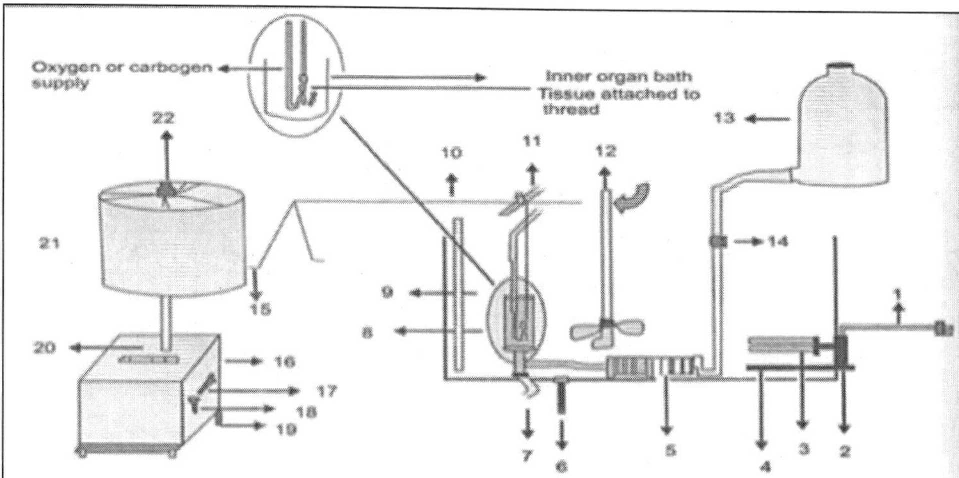

1. Power input
2. Switch board
3. Heating rod
4. Thermostat
5. Coiled PSS inlet to inner bath
6. Outer bath water outlet
7. Inner bath PSS outlet
8. Inner bath with air supply (aerator) and tissue holder
9. Thermometer
10. Recording lever
11. Fulcrum
12. Stirrer
13. Reservoir for PSS
14. Clip to control the flow of PSS to inner bath
15. Stylus or writing point
16. Motor
17. Gear to adjust the speed
18. Clutch lever
19. Screw to adjust the level of drum
20. Drum rotation indicator
21. Sherrington rotating drum
22. Lift screw (to move drum up or down)

Figure 6.1: Diagrammatic Representation of a Typical Organ Bath.

1. **Outer bath/Outer water jacket:** It is made up of steel or Perspex glass. It remains filled with water. It is used to store water outside the inner organ bath to maintain the temperature for the experiment.
2. **Inner organ bath:** The tissue under study is kept inside and it consisting of glass PSS.
3. **Water heater/heating coil:** It is fitted in outer organ bath and heat the water.
4. **Thermostat:** As the name suggests, it is a temperature regulating device that maintains a constant temperature of water in the outer organ bath.
5. **Rotator/Stirrer:** It causes circulation of water in outer organ bath and maintains the uniform temperature throughout the outer organ bath.
6. **Mariotte bottle/Aspiration bottle:** It acts as a reservoir for PSS. It delivers a constant rate of flow from closed bottles.
7. **Areator cum tissue holder tube:** It provides continuous air or oxygen supply to the tissue and also holds the tissue.
8. **Fulcrum:** Writing lever is attached to this and helps in a free vertical movement to record the response.
9. **Pre heating coil:** Maintains temperature of PSS when outer organ bath is empty.

10. **Recording lever:** It is a mechanical part made up of aluminium and steel. It is light in weight and very strong so that it do not bend while writing on a smoked surface.
11. **Kymograph:** It is an electrical part used to record the response of the tissue. Its various parts are a rotating drum, base and shaft.
    - I) **Rotating drum:** It rotates in a clockwise direction so that it can be read from left to right. Also known as Sherrington Rotating drum. Its speed can be adjusted by the attached lever and gear. Kymogram is the paper wrapped around the drum to record the response.
    - II) **Base:** Made up of lever and gear.
    - III) **Shaft:** Shaft is the elongated part having a screw to adjust the level of the drum.

Smoking of Kymograph drum: After fixing of paper to the drum it should be smoked properly with the help of burning cotton soaked in kerosene.

Fixing of the tracings: Recordings on the smoked drum are preserved by fixing.

Selection of tissue for organ bath: There is a diverse range of tissue preparations that can be studied in vitro using organ bath experiments. The majority of organs in the body contain muscle cells which contract as part of their normal physiology. Specific preparations have become associated with a certain type of physiological or pharmacological investigation. Preparations are selected on the basis of whether they express the receptor or response of interest and the ease with which other techniques can be used in combination. The species used will also be an important consideration, as the degree of homology with human physiology varies between species. There are also species-specific advantages and disadvantages associated with the same

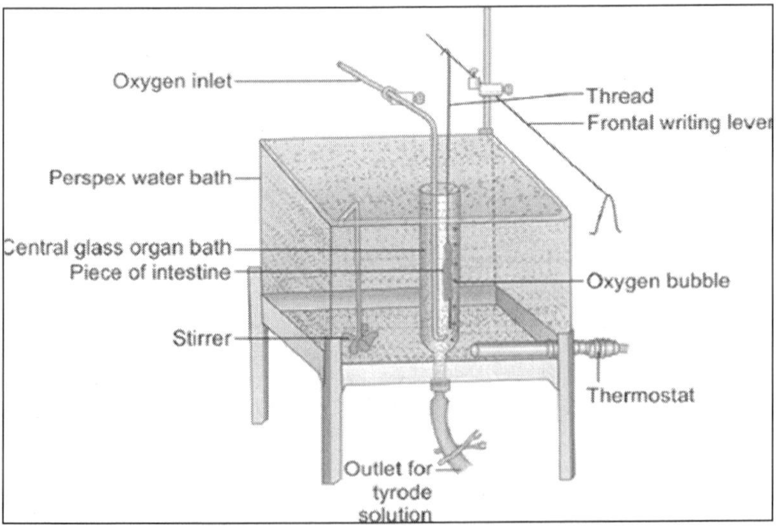

Figure 6.2: Systematic Arrangement of Tissue Organ Bath.
(*Source*: Geetha N, 2017. Practical Physiology, Jaypee Digital Publisher. DOI- 10.5005/jp/books/12995_54).

tissue type. For example, the guinea pig ileum is an excellent tissue to study the actions of drugs targeting the parasympathetic nervous system and gastrointestinal physiology and pharmacology. In contrast, the rat ileum is difficult to use in the isolated set-up as it contracts spontaneously, interfering with drug-induced effects. Part of the decision about which tissue to use may be whether to provide exogenous electrical stimulation. When the tissue is removed from the animal, the neuronal input from the central nervous system (CNS) and periphery is severed, but the nerve terminals remain and neurotransmitter release can be elicited by applying electrical stimulation. In the case of the parasympathetic nervous system, the ganglion is also present in some isolated tissue preparations, *e.g.* isolated guinea pig ileum. Another commonly used stimulated tissue preparation is the vas deferens, which provides a useful tissue for studying the sympathetic nervous system.

Physiological Salt Solution

According to **different tissue** to be used, there is a **different physiological solution** prepared. Different organic salts are used in preparation of PSS, these salts all together provide an artificial media resembling inorganic composition to blood plasma. But all or most of them contain the following ingredients at different concentrations:

Table 6.1: Composition of different Physiological Salt Solution (Salt in g/10 Liters)

Ingredient	*Frog Ringer Solution*	*Kreb's Solution*	*Tyrode Solution*	*Ringer Locke Solution*	*De Jalon Solution*	*Mc Ewen Solution*
NaCl	65	69	80	91.5	90	76
KCl	1.4	3.5	2.0	4.2	4.2	4.2
$MgCl_{2.}6H_2O$	-	1.1	1.0	-	-	-
$NaH_2Po_{4.}H_2O$	0.1	1.4	0.5			1.4
$NaHCO_3$	2	21	10	1.5	5	21
$CaCl_2$	1.2	2.8	2.0	2.4	0.6	2.4
Glucose	20	20	10	10	5	20
Aerating Gas	Air	O_2+5%Co_2	O_2 or Air	Pure O_2	O_2+5%Co_2	O_2+5%Co_2

1. **Nacl** → to adjust the isotonicity.
2. **Glucose** → nutrient.
3. **Ca+2, K+, sometimes Mg+2 as CL salt** ≡ to maintain normal muscle contraction.
4. **Sodium bicarbonate** → to adjust pH similar to that of blood.
5. **NaH_2PO_4** (sodium di hydrogen phosphate) buffer→ to compensate for any change in pH.

Table 6.2: Examples of Tissues Commonly Used in the Organ Bath Set-up and their Associated Pharmacology

Sl. No.	Tissue type	Commonly Used Animal Species	Concerned Pharmacology
1.	**Ileum (Small intestine)** Nicotinic and muscarinic cholinergic receptors (Contract) Histamine receptors (Contract)	Guinea pig	Parasympathetic innervations (Electrically evoked neuro-transmitter release inhibited by opioid receptors)
2.	**Bladder** Beta-adrenoceptors (relax)	Guinea pig, rat and mouse	Muscarinic receptors (Contract)
3.	**Aorta** Beta-adrenoceptors (relax) Alpha$_1$-adrenoceptors and 5-HT receptors (contract)	Guinea pig, rat and mouse (difficult)	Muscarinic receptors (Contract)
4.	**Heart** Beta-adrenoceptors (increase force and rate)	Guinea pig, rat and mouse	Muscarinic receptors (slow force and rate)
5.	**Uterus** Beta-adrenoceptors (relax) Histamine receptors (Relax)	Rat	Muscarinic receptors (Contract)
6.	**Vas deferens** Alpha$_1$-adrenoceptors (contract)	Rat, mouse	Sympathetic innervations (Electrically evoked neuro-transmitter release inhibited by Alpha$_2$-adrenoceptors receptors)
7.	**Tracheal spiral** Beta-adrenoceptors(relax) **Gastric fundus (Part of stomach)** 5-HT receptors (contract)	Guinea pig and RatRat	Muscarinic receptors (Contract) muscarinic receptors (Contract)
8.	**Isolated nerve**	Frog	Na^+ and K^+ channels (Local anesthetics block action potential)

The two most commonly used physiological solutions are **Tyrode's** and **Krebs.**

Tyrode's Solution

It is a solution that is roughly isotonic with interstitial fluid and used in physiological experiments and tissue culture. It resembles lactated Ringer's solution, but contains magnesium, a sugar (usually glucose) as an energy source and uses bicarbonate and phosphate as a buffer instead of lactate. Some variations also include phosphate and sulfate ions. It must be gassed with 95 per cent oxygen and N2, 5 per cent carbon dioxide when used for cell culture applications and physiology experiments in order to achieve an appropriate pH. With the addition of extra potassium salt, it can be used to prepare a cardioplegic solution[7].

Krebs Solution

It contains Sodium (Na), Potassium (K), Chloride (Cl),Calcium (Ca), Magnesium sulfate ($MgSO_4$), bicarbonate (HCO_3), Phosphate (PO_4), glucose, albumin and tromethamine(THAM).It is used for studying arteries ex vivo and during isolated muscle testing of mammalian skeletal muscles[8].

Aeration

Physiological salt solutions should be aerated by a suitable gas:

1. Pure oxygen → for heart tissues.
2. Normal air → for intestine.
3. Carbogen (95 per cent O_2, 5 per cent CO_2) → used for uterus.

Temperature

Mammalian tissue must be bathed in a warmed solution adjusted at 37°C *e.g.* Isolated rabbit intestine.The temperature should be decreased in some experiments to reduce the myogenic contraction, the warmed solution adjusted at 32°C *e.g.* Guinea-pig ileum. Amphibian tissues survive at room temperature (25°C) *e.g.* frog rectus abdominis.

Limitations of Isolated Tissue and Organ Preparations

Difficulty in exactly maintain the normal physiological environment of the test sample. If a tissue is not perfused through its blood vessels or is not porous, the oxygen delivery and nutrients is restricted by diffusion. Some tissue requires high oxygen and nutrient consumption, such as cardiac muscle, a hypoxic core may exist if the tissue is >0.5mm thick. If the tissue size is not thin, the requirements of nutrients and oxygen must be low, as in the case of smooth muscle. Other problems may arise due to imbalances in oncotic pressure or trace elements caused by the use of media, overstretching, mechanical damage to cell layers. When used these limitations in mind, the tissue organ bath system is a very useful screening and research tools.

REFERENCES

1. Emma Robinson Physiology and Pharmacology, University of Bristol, UK.
2. Pharmacological Experiments on Isolated Preparations, second edition. E and S Livingstone, Edinburgh. Kitchen, I (1984).
3. Textbook of *in vitro* Practical Pharmacology. Blackwell Scientific Publications, Oxford.
4. Laboratory practical to study the differential innervation pathways of urinary tract smooth muscle Benjamin E. Rembetski, Caroline A. Cobine, and X Bernard T. Drumm Department of Physiology and Cell Biology, University of Nevada, Reno School of Medicine, Reno, Nevada. 2018.
5. Fully Automated Experiments with Isolated Organs In Vitro JOOP S. DE GRAAF, COR J. DE Vos, AND HANS J. STEENBERGEN

6. Brit. J. Pharmacol. (1964)) 23, 360-373. THE USE OF ISOLATED ORGANS FOR DETECTING ACTIVE SUBSTANCES IN THE CIRCULATING BLOOD BY J. R. VANE From the Department of Pharmacology, Institute of Basic Medical Sciences, Royal College of Surgeons of England, Lincoln's Inn Fields, London, W.C.2

7. Tyrode, M.V. (1910) Arch. Int. Pharmacodyn. Ther. 20: 205

8. Methods in Pharmacology Volume 3 Smooth muscle. Eds. E.E. Daniel and D.M. Paton PlenumPress, NY, 1975.

Chapter 7

General Diagnostic Toxicology

Diagnosis depends heavily on a systematic approach that includes proper sample collection and handling. Such cases require piecing together a "diagnostic puzzle" that includes a complete case history, clinical signs, clinicopathologic findings, postmortem findings, results from chemical analyses and occasionally bioassay findings.

History

The primary goal of the history is to identify possible sources of a toxicant. Sources are found by examining the environment, reviewing management practices, and recording the movement and fate of animals, feed, water, and bedding. The investigation of the individual animals should review the history of vaccinations, feeding, onset of signs, specificity of signs, severity, and progression of signs, and response to treatment. Recent medication history should be recorded, including information about the substances given, time of administration, amount and reasons for use, and individuals treating the animal.

Sample Collect and Storage

Samples for toxicology testing fall into three general categories: environmental, antemortem and postmortem.

- ☆ **ENVIRONMENTAL SAMPLES:** Many toxicants are not detectable in tissues. Thus, environmental samples (*e.g.*, source materials, feeds) are critical to diagnosis in a poisoning case as well as being important for identifying and removing the source of poison.
- ☆ **FEED SAMPLES**: To avoid dilution, samples should not be pooled between lots, shipments, feed bunks, or animal pens. Pooling is desirable, however, if done within the same lot of feed or stack of hay from one field to ensure that the sample is representative of the lot. For example,

mold toxins (*e.g.*, aflatoxin in grain or nitrate from weeds) in a lot of hay occur in "hot spots," or isolated portions of a lot or bag. Thus, one grab sample from one part of a bin may miss the toxin, but multiple samples from different parts of the bin have a greater chance of locating the toxin. Samples are individually labeled. Sample sizes vary, but the optimal size in most instances is about 500 g of material (about 1 lb). Some samples may be considerably larger to ensure adequate representation of the lot in question. Moist samples should be frozen. Feeds to be kept dry should be stored in a cool, dry environment in containers that discourage condensation and mold growth (plastic bags promote decay).

- ☆ **WATER SAMPLES** Water samples are obtained at the source (well, canal, pond), in transit (piping, tankers), in storage tanks, and at the site of exposure. Spills are sampled if animals are exposed to the materials. The history should include recent occurrences regarding the water (tides, storage). Some chemicals are toxic in water, even when present in very low concentrations. Thus, two 1-L samples should be obtained from each site. Glass preserving jars (1 L) are useful for water samples. Plastic and metal containers should be avoided. Metal and salt samples can be covered with plastic wrap and then the lid; organic chemical samples should be covered with foil and then the lid. For extremely sensitive tests, the jars can be rinsed with acetone (nail polish remover) and then the source water itself before filling with the sample. Small samples of blue-green algae can be mixed half and half with 10 per cent neutral buffered formalin for identification, with larger samples (up to 5 gallons) being saved in plastic buckets for possible toxin identification using bioassay or instrumental techniques.
- ☆ **PLANT SAMPLES:** Many plant poisonings still rely on plant identification for diagnosis. Pastures should be examined, with plants being identified as the investigation proceeds. Grabbing a single flake of hay at random and sending for plant identification is usually unrewarding. Several bales should be opened until suspicious weeds are found (if present). The amount of the weeds in the bale, stack, or lot should be estimated, and then the weeds can be sent to a laboratory for identification if needed. Assistance with the identification of plants can be found from a number of sources. Occasionally, a specialist from a herbarium or agricultural extension can be found to walk a field. If local experts are available, representative specimens of fresh plants (including flower, greenery, and roots) are obtained, wrapped with wet newspaper, and taken for identification. If local help is unavailable, samples can be catalogued pressed in folds of newspaper under heavy books, and then shipped to a diagnostic service for identification. Rapid plant identifications can be attempted by pressing a plant on a high-quality office copier and transmitting the copy by FAX for identification.

Identification of a potentially toxic plant is not usually definitive; it only suggests an opportunity for exposure. Diagnosis of plant poisoning also requires evidence of the consumption of a plant by the animal. That evidence may include an abundance of the plant in the field, indications of grazing (stripped stalks or topped plants).

Suspected Poison	*Required Material in Order of Importance*
Arsenic (Acute)	Liver, kidneys, stomach contents
Arsenic (Chronic)	Hair, liver, urine
Alkaloids	Liver, urine, brain, stomach contents.
Copper	Liver
Cyanide (HCN)	Stomach contents, liver, oxalated blood
Chlorinated insecticides	Fat, liver, stomach contents
OPC	Oxalated blood, whole blood, stomach contents
Lead (Acute)	Kidney, Liver, urine
Lead (Chronic)	Hair, liver, kidneys, urine
Mercury	Liver, kidney, stomach contents, intestinal contents
Nitrate/nitrite	Stomach contents, whole blood
Phosphorous	Stomach contents, Liver, oxalated blood
Phenol – cresols	Liver, stomach contents, kidney
Rodenticides	Stomach contents, liver, urine
Strychnine	Stomach contents, urine, liver, brain, kidneys
Sodium chloride	Oxalated whole blood brain, stomach contents, liver

Blood	30 to 50 ml	**Kidneys**	One
Brain	Entire	**Liver**	500-1000 g
Fat	200 gm	**Stomach contents**	500 – 1000g in LA and available contents in small animal
Hair	5- 10 gm	**Urine**	All available
Intestinal contents	500-1000 g		

Detection of Hydrocyanic Acid

A) Qualitative Test

Steyn Test

Take the suspected sample (finely chopped plant content/rumen content) in a test tube add few drops of chloroform and water. Insert a piece of moistened sodium picrate paper at the mouth of tube with a cork (paper should not touch the sample). Incubate the test tube overnight at 37^0 C. The gradual turning of paper into orange and then brick red confirms the presence of cyanogenetic glycosides or HCN in the sample.

Dry materials like seeds should be grounded and moistened with water and allowed to hydrolyse in a test tube containing sodium picrate paper and incubated at 37 to 39^{0}C overnight.

Colour Tests Methods[6]

Prussian Blue Test

Prepare a concentrated alkaline solution of the sample by heating it in a water bath. To 2 mL of this solution, add few drops of freshly prepared 5 per cent solution of Ferrous Sulphate and 1 drop of Ferric Chloride solution. Heat the mixture just by boiling and simultaneously add dilute sulphuric acid dropwise to the solution slightly acidic.

The formation of Prussian blue colour indicates the presence of hydrocyanic acid. A precipitate may be observed on keeping the content undisturbed overnight[2].

B) Quantitative Test

Acid-titration Method

Mix 10-20 grams of suspected sample (finely chopped plant material/rumen content) in 100 ml of water in a Kjeldahl flask and macerate at room temperature for 100 to 120 minutes. Add 100 ml of water and steam distil, collecting distillate in 0.02 N $AgNO_3$, acidified with 1mL HNO_3. Collect 150 mL of distillate and filtered through gooch crucible. Both the receiver and gooch crucible are washed with a small amount of H_2O_2. Excess $AgNO_3$ in the filter is tittered using ferric alum as an indicator.

1 mL of 0.02 N $AgNO_3$ = 0.54 mg of HCN

Detection of Thiocyanates

Qualitative Test

Add 0.1 ml of ferric chloride solution to 0.1 mL of sample and mix. A deep red colour indicates the presence of thiocyanate.

Detection of Alkaloids

A) Qualitative Test

The suspected sample (plant material/liver and stomach/intestinal or rumen content) is extracted refluxly with alcohol on a hot water bath for an hour, cooled and filtered. The extracted alcoholic extract is dried on a porcelain dish on a water bath. Diluted Hydrochloric acid is used to dissolve the dried residue, which is further filtered using filter paper.

The supernatant is precipitated with ammonia and alkaloid is extracted with 20 mL chloroform in a separating funnel. The chloroform extract is separated, evaporated and extracted on a watch glass which is further acidified with HCl. One or two drops of Mayer's reagent or Dragandroff's reagent are placed separately on the watch glass and are allowed to mix by diffusion.

The presence of alkaloids in the suspected sample is indicated by white precipitate at the junction of two solutions.

B) Quantitative Test

Prolius Fluid Method

Dried powdered plant of known quantity is soaked overnight in prolius fluid. The supernatant is emptied and fresh prolius fluid is added and again left overnight. The same process is repeated 3-4 times so that all alkaloid residue is extracted. The combined extract is concentrated at low temperature, and different fractions of solvents *i.e.*, ether (30-40^{0}C), Chloroform (60-65^{0}C) and alcohol (80^{0}C) are distilled separately. The concentrated extract is again treated 2-3 times with 10 per cent HCl. The resulted concentrated extract is extracted further with petroleum ether (to remove the oily substances).

Ammonia is added to the extract to make it alkaline and extracted with chloroform. The extract is then washed 2-3 times with water and concentrated by distillation. The extract is completely dried and weighed to determine the quantity of the alkaloid.

Detection of Strychnine

Spot Test

About 2-3 ml of suspected sample (stomach contents/urine/serum) is taken in a clean and dry test tube. Concentrated sulphuric acid (5 ml) is added into the test tube and stirred well with a glass rod. A few crystals of potassium dichromate are added to the tube and mixed well.

The tube is then examined in front of the light. The appearance of falling streamers of blue, violet, red and orange indicate the presence of strychnine.

Confirmatory Test

This test is applicable to stomach content and scene residues. In a clean, dry test tube 1 ml of each sample and concentrated hydrochloric acid are added respectively. A granule of Zinc is added to the test tube and the tube is then heated in a water bath for 10 mins.

Any remaining zinc is removed after cooling the test tube and 50 µl of sodium nitrite solution is added to it. The presence of pink colour confirms strychnine in the sample. The sensitivity of this test for strychnine is 10 mg/L.

Sunshine Method

Weigh 5 gm suspected sample (feed or stomach/rumen contents) and add 10 N NaOH to it. In case if the suspected sample is a tissue sample, homogenize 5 gm sample and make it alkaline with 10 N NaOH. Transfer to seperatory funnel and shake with 100 ml chloroform. To 80 ml of chloroform extract add 5 ml of 0.1 N H_2SO_4 and then made alkaline with 10 N NaOH. Re extract with chloroform, filter the chloroform layer and evaporate to dryness. Redissolve the residue in 0.1 ml ethanol and spot on the TLC plate. Develop the plate in a mixture of solvent containing chloroform: acetone-50:50. Remove the plate, dry and spray with Dragendorff's reagent. Strychnine appears at Rf value of 0.75.

Test for Tannins

Diluted aqueous extract of the sample turns green or bluish with the addition of $FeCl_2$ solution in the presence of tannins.

10 gm of finely grounded material (oil cakes/concentrate mixture) in a separating funnel and soaked completely with ethyl alcohol and wait for 5 mins. First drop of solvent extract is collected on a filter paper and dried completely. A drop of Antimony trichloride solution (prepared in chloroform) is put over it. The paper is heated gently on a spirit lamp without charring. The appearance of pink colour indicates the presence of Mohua saponin[3].

Detection of Oxalate Poisoning

In a test tube, take 1 ml clear stomach contents or urine and add 0.2 ml concentrated ammonium hydroxide and heat it on flame of a burner or spirit lamp to evaporate the solution. Add 40 mg thiobarbituric acid crystals and gently reheat on burner or spirit lamp. Formation of an orange red colour, which is soluble in ethanol indicative of oxalates in the samples.

Qualitative Test

Mix 1 ml of calcium chloride solution and add 2ml of clear test solution. Add 1 ml of Acetic acid, if precipitate forms. The white precipitate which is insoluble in acetic acid indicates the presence of oxalate, fluoride or Sulphate.

If precipitate still remains, centrifuge the solution and add 1 ml of dil. Hydrochloric acid. If the precipitate obtained above is soluble in hydrochloric acid, oxalate is present[4].

Estimation of Nitrate/Nitrite

Qualitative Test

- Plant material is extracted using pestle mortar with water, and rumen contents can be filtered. A small quantity of plant extract/suspected material is put on a clean dry slab, and 1-2 drops of 1 per cent solution of diphenylamine in concentrated H_2SO_4 solution are added close to it and allowed to mix via diffusion. A blue ring formation at the junction indicates the presence of nitrate/nitrite.
- In case of grinded fodder or feed, add 5-10 ml of distilled water along with 5 gm of suspected sample in a beaker and mix well. Keep the solution for 30 mins and then centrifuge it. Take 2 ml of supernatant in the test tube and add 2 ml of sulfanilic acid in 20 per cent glacial acetic acid. Add 2 ml of 0.15 per cent alpha-napthylamine hydrochloride in 20 per cent glacial acetic acid. Pink to red colour development indicates the presence of nitrate in the sample.

- ☆ Centrifuge the suspected clear stomach/intestinal content or urine. Add 0.1 ml of it in a test tube containing 0.1 ml sulfanilic acid and mix well. Add 0.1 ml imipramine solution and 0.2 ml concentration H_2SO_4. Development of blue colour indicates the presence of nitrate in the sample.

Quantitative Estimation of Nitrites

Fine powdered sample (100 gm) is taken and oven dried, which is then transferred into a beaker. Now 9 ml of silver Sulphate solution is added, swirled quickly and immediately 1 ml of sodium phosphate solution is added, which precipitates the excess silver. The solution is left undisturbed for 2 hours and then filtered using filter paper No. 42.

Add 2 ml of Copper Sulphate solution to the equal amount of filtrate and water[5].

Estimation of Nitrites

Dissolve 3.3 gm of sulphanlinic acid 750 ml of water and 250 ml of glacial acetic acid. In another flask boil 0.5 gm of alpha- napthylamine in 100 ml. Take 1 ml of this extract in 50 ml volumetric flask. Add 40 ml of distilled water and then 2 ml of solution.

Spot Test for Nitrite Poisoning

- ☆ Take 1 ml clear stomach contents or urine in a test tube and add 0.1 ml imipramine solution. Mix well.
- ☆ Add 0.2 ml hydrochloric acid. The development of blue colour in the tube is indicative of nitrite in the sample

Estimation of Nitrite in Blood and Urine

- ☆ Blood, serum, and urinary nitrite are estimated by Griess reaction

Reagents Required

- ☆ $ZnSO_4$ Solution: 75 mM/L in distilled water
- ☆ NaOH reagent 55 mM/L in distilled water.
- ☆ Griess reagent: Made 1 sulfanilamide, 0.2 per cent naphthalene diamine hydrochloride and 2.5 per cent phosphoric acid.
- ☆ Standard $KMnO_4$ solution make different concentrations

Procedure

- ☆ Blood/serum (2 ml) is subjected to deproteinization by adding 2 ml $ZnSO_4$ Solution and 2 ml NaOH reagent. Allow to stand for 10 min and centrifuge or filter.
- ☆ Take 1 ml of deproteinized sample or 1 ml urine sample, 1 ml of standard and 1 ml deionized water in tubes marked as a sample, standard and blank, respectively. Take different concentrations of standard.

- ☆ Add 1 ml Griess reagent and mix.
- ☆ Incubate the tubes at room temperature for 15 min. Measure the absorbance at 545 nm against blank.
- ☆ Standard curve is prepared with known concentration of sodium nitrite Extrapolate the value of nitrite in the sample from the standard graph.

REFERENCES

1. Singh, H.B., Wasi, N. and Mehra, M.C., 1986. Detection and determination of cyanide- a review. *International journal of environmental analytical chemistry*, 26 **(2),** p.115.
2. Fear, C.M., 1929. The alkaloid test for tannins. *Analyst*, *54***(639)**, pp.316-318.
3. https: //www.who.int/ipcs/publications/training_poisons/basic_analytical_tox/en/index6.html
4. Hassan, S.S.M., 1973. New spot tests for nitrates and nitrites. *Microchemical Journal*, *18*(5), pp.486-490.
5. West, P.W. and Sarma, P.L., 1957. A spot test for nitrates. *Microchimica Acta*, *45*(3-4), pp.506-509.

Chapter 8

Reproductive and Developmental Toxicity Assessment

Reproductive toxicology is the subject area dealing with the causes, mechanisms, effects and prevention of disturbances throughout the entire reproductive cycle, including infertility induced by chemicals. It also includes the harmful effects of agents on progeny and/or impairment of male and female reproductive functions. Additional studies should be conducted in conjunction with reproductive toxicology studies to determine whether the drug is teratogenic or has an effect on perinatal/ postnatal development. These studies should also investigate the drug's potential effects on fertility and reproductive performance. These studies are divided into two categories: reproductive and developmental toxicology studies. Adverse effects on the developing organism caused by exposure prior to conception, during the prenatal period, or after birth until sexual maturity are referred to as developmental toxicity.

Reproduction and Development Toxicity Studies

A three-segment testing protocol has been used in most reproductive studies in which both male and female rats are studied in segment I for fertility and general reproductive performance. Segment II includes teratology or embryo-fetal toxicity studies in rats and rabbits whereas segment III includes perinatal and postnatal development studies in rats to assess drug effects during the third trimester of pregnancy and lactation.

The following are the most common manifestations of reproductive and developmental toxicity studies:

1. Reproductive toxicity in both male and female
2. Pregnancy
3. Lactation

4. Mortality
5. Dysmorphogenesis (Structural abnormalities)
6. Growth Modifications
7. Disturbance in Functioning

Protocols for Laboratory Testing

The procedures to be used to provide data for risk assessments are described in testing protocols. The design and execution of the tests, including endpoint selection and resolving power, determine the quality and utility of the data. A single protocol is unlikely to contain all of the information needed to conduct a comprehensive risk assessment. For example, the test design required to determining the reversibility of adverse effects or the mechanism of toxic action may differ from that required to determine the time of onset of an effect or to calculate a safe level for long-term repeated exposure. When performing a risk assessment, results from several different types of tests should be available. In most cases, only a limited amount of information is available. In those circumstances, the limited data should be used to assess risk to the greatest extent possible. The evaluations of the protocols from which data are available, as well as the quality of the resulting data, are essential parts of the hazard characterization and quantitative dose-response processes. Design factors that are particularly important in reproductive toxicity testing are discussed in this section. Following that, standardized protocols are described that may provide useful data for reproductive risk assessments.

Dosing Interval

A prolonged treatment period is required to appropriately evaluate the potential effects of an agent on the reproductive systems. For example, damage to spermatogonial stem cells, will not appear in cauda epididymis or ejaculate samples for 8 to 14 weeks, depending on the test species. The suitability of the dosing duration is a critical factor in risk assessment in some situations like, with some chemical agents that bio-accumulate, the full impact on a given cell type, as well as the impact on functional endpoints like fertility, could be delayed even further.

On the other hand, adaptation may occur, allowing tolerance to levels of a chemical that previously caused an adverse effect. A good example is chlordimeform's interference with ovulation which has a compensatory mechanism. [1] In this case the compensatory mechanism can thus be activated with continued dosing and masking the initial adverse effect. Knowledge of relevant pharmacokinetic and pharmacodynamics data can help with dose selection and treatment duration in these situations. The proper timing of examination of treated animals in relation to the initiation and termination of exposure to the agent is also critical.

Duration of Mating

Traditionally, male and female rats or mice are allowed to put together for a period of time ranging from a few days to three weeks. Given a four or five day estrous cycle, each female should be in estrus four or five times during a twenty one day mating period if she is cycling normally. As a result, data on the number of cycles or intervals required to achieve pregnancy may provide evidence of reduced fertility that is not available from fertility data. Furthermore, the male has the opportunity to copulate multiple times during each period of behavioral estrus, resulting in the delivery of far more sperm than is required for fertilization. When fertility testing allows an unlimited number of mattings, a significant impact on sperm production is required before an adverse effect on fertility can be detected.

Number of Females Mated to each Male

In the multigeneration reproduction test, the EPA test guidelines prepared pursuant to FIFRA and TSCA, specify the use of 20 males and enough females to produce at least 20 pregnancies for each dose group in each generation. [2-4] However, 20 pregnancies may have been achieved in some tests that did not follow EPA test guidelines by mating two females with each male and using fewer than 20 males per treatment group. In such cases, the data's statistical treatment should be carefully scrutinized. The degree of independence of the observations for each female may not be known when multiple females are mated to each male. When the cause of an adverse effect cannot be assigned to only one sex with certainty, dependence should be assumed and the male used as the experimental unit in statistical analyses. The ability to detect an effect is reduced when the experimental unit consists of fewer males.

Reproduction Tests for Single and Multiple Generations

Continuous exposure to a test substance for one or more generations is common in reproductive toxicity studies in laboratory animals. The goal is to detect and study effects on the entire reproductive process as well as the individual reproductive organs. The Agency, in accordance with FIFRA and TSCA, as well as the OECD, has published test guidelines for single and multi-generation reproduction protocols [5, 6]. The single-generation reproduction test assesses the effects of peripubertal and adult animals being exposed to sub chronic radiation. Whereas F1 and F2 offspring are exposed continuously in utero from conception to birth, as well as during the pre-weaning period, in the multigenerational reproduction protocol. This allows for the detection of effects that occur as a result of exposures at various stages of development, including puberty and young adulthood. Because the parental and subsequent filial generations have different exposure histories, the reproductive effects observed in one generation may not be comparable to those observed in another. Furthermore, due to factors such as continued parental exposure, increased parental age, sexual experience, and female parity, successive litters from the same parents cannot be considered replicates.

Rats are commonly used in single-generation and multigenerational reproduction tests. Dosing is started at five to eight weeks of age and continued for eight to ten weeks prior to mating in a typical reproduction test to allow gametogenesis effects to be expressed and increase the likelihood of detecting histologic lesions. Typically, three dose levels and one or more control groups are included. For each generation, enough males and females are mated to ensure twenty pregnancies per dose group.

The first generation of offspring should be referred to as the parental (P) generation, with all subsequent generations being referred to as filial generations (F_1, F_2). In a single-generation test, only the P generation is mated, whereas in a two-generation test, both the P and F_1 generations are mated. Both females and males in the P generation are treated prior to and during mating, with treatment typically beginning around puberty. Cohabitation can last up to three weeks during which time the females are checked for signs of mating. During pregnancy and lactation, females are still exposed [3].

After weaning (day 21) and through the mating period, randomly selected F1 male and female offspring are exposed in the two-generation reproduction test. Mated F1 females are treated throughout their pregnancy and lactation. From either P or F1 animals, more than one litter can be produced. It is important to consider that offspring may be exposed to a chemical through ingestion of maternal feed or water (diet or drinking water studies), licking of exposed fur (inhalation study), contact with treated skin (dermal study), or coprophagia, as well as through the milk, depending on the route of exposure of lactating females.

Visual examination of the reproductive organs is usually one of the reproductive endpoints evaluated in P and F generations in single- and multigenerational reproduction tests. Males' testes, epididymis, and accessory sex glands' weights and histopathology may be available, while females' vagina, uterus, cervix, ovaries, and mammary glands' histopathology may be available. Weights of the uterus and ovaries are frequently available. Furthermore, litters are weighed at birth and examined for the number of live and dead offspring, gender, gross abnormalities, growth, and weaning survival.

If the only negative effects observed in a study using one of these protocols are effects on fertility or pregnancy outcome, the contributions of male- and female-specific effects are often difficult to differentiate. It may be possible to characterize a male-specific effect if testicular histopathology or sperm evaluations are included. Similarly, changes in estrous cycle normality or ovarian and reproductive tract histology could indicate female-specific effects. However, the presence of effects in one sex does not rule out the possibility that both sexes were negatively affected. A one-generation study is insufficient for identifying all potential reproductive toxicants because it would oversight the effects caused by prenatal and postnatal exposures, as well as effects on germ cells that could be passed down and expressed in the next generation [7]. Because of the shorter duration of exposure for the P generation, a one-generation test may oversight adverse effects with delayed or latent onset. These limitations apply to both the longer-term "screening" protocols and the shorter-term "screening" protocols. Because of these limitations, the results of a two-generation test or its equivalent should be included in a comprehensive reproductive risk assessment. Also sperm analysis and estrous cycle normality be included as endpoints in reproductive effects studies. In the proposed revisions to the EPA test guideline; these endpoints have been included [4].

Alternative Tests for Reproductive Health

There have been several shorter-term reproductive toxicity screening tests developed. The reproductive/developmental toxicity screening test [8-10], a tripartite protocol developed by the international conference on harmonization [11, 12] and the reproductive/developmental toxicity screening test [8, 13]. These protocols were created to help determine which tests should be prioritized for further testing and should not be used to determine regulatory exposure levels. Because of their short exposure periods, they are unable to assess certain aspects of the reproductive process that are covered by multigenerational reproduction protocols, such as developmentally induced effects on offspring's reproductive systems.

The **male dominant lethal test** was designed to identify mutagenic effects in the male spermatogenic process that are fatal to offspring. To detect equivalent effects on oogenesis, a **female dominant lethal protocol** was also used [14]. Acute dosing (1 to 5 days) followed by serial mattings with one or two females per male per week for the duration of the spermatogenic process may be used in dominant lethal protocols. Sub chronic dosing for the duration of the spermatogenic process, followed by mating, is an alternative protocol. The acute protocol's dose levels are usually higher than the sub chronic protocol's dose levels. Females are monitored for signs of mating, sacrificed around the midpoint of pregnancy, and examined for pre- and post-implantation loss.

An acute exposure protocol combined with serial mating could help to figure out which spermatogenic cell types are affected by treatment. On the other hand, acute dosing may not produce adverse effects at levels as low as sub-chronic dosing due to factors like bioaccumulation. In contrast, if tolerance to an agent develops over time, an effect may be observed after a single dose that is not detected after repeated doses.

Sub chronic toxicity tests may have been performed prior to the start of a comprehensive reproduction study. Exposure to rats in a sub-chronic toxicity test usually begins at six- eight weeks of age and lasts for ninety days [2, 3], allowing the animals to reach a more mature stage of sexual development and ensuring an adequate length of dosing for most agents to observe effects on the reproductive organs. Oral or gavage administration is common, but dermal or inhalation administration is also possible. Throughout the test, the animals are monitored for clinical signs and are sacrificed at the end of dosing.

Visual examination of the reproductive organs, as well as weights and histopathology for the testes, epididymis, and accessory sex glands, are common endpoints for the male reproductive system whereas visual examination of the reproductive organs, uterine and ovarian weights, and histopathology of the vagina, uterus, cervix, ovaries, and mammary glands may be used as endpoints in females. This test may be useful in identifying a potential reproductive hazard, but it typically does not provide information about the integrated function of the reproductive systems (sexual behaviour, fertility, and pregnancy outcomes), nor does it include effects on immature animals.

Chronic toxicity tests allowed assessing the harmful effects of long-term exposures. Soon after weaning, oral, inhalation, or dermal exposure is started and it is usually continued for twelve to twenty four months. Males have their reproductive organs visually examined, their testes weighed, and their testes and accessory sex glands histopathological examined. In females, the reproductive organs are visually examined, uterine and ovarian weights are obtained, and the reproductive organs are histopathological evaluated. In the reproductive tracts of aged control animals, the incidence of pathologic conditions is frequently increased. As a result, findings should be interpreted with caution.

Test Species Endpoints for Evaluating Male and Female Reproductive Toxicity

Introduction

The endpoints of reproductive toxicity are divided into three categories in these Guidelines: couple-mediated, male-specific and female-specific. Couple-mediated endpoints are those where both sexes can play a role if both partners are exposed. As a result, exposure to either sex or both sexes could have an impact on that endpoint. Results should be evaluated on a case-by-case basis with all of the evidence considered. Scientific judgment should be used extensively. All effects that may be considered as adverse are appropriate for use in establishing a NOAEL, LOAEL, or benchmark dose.

Couple-mediated Endpoints

The most comprehensive and direct insight into reproductive capability comes from data on fertility potential and associated reproductive outcomes. As previously stated, most protocols only allow exposed males to live with exposed females. This makes resolving gender-specific influences more difficult. Conclusions may need to be limited to noting that when one or both parents are potentially exposed, the "couple" is at reproductive risk.

Fertility and Reproductive Outcomes

Breeding studies with test species provide a wealth of information on reproductive toxins. Fertility and pregnancy test results are used to assess the functional consequences of reproductive injury. The Agency's Guidelines for Developmental Toxicity Risk Assessment list and discuss a number of endpoints that are relevant to developmental toxicity [15].

Table 8.1: Endpoints of Reproductive Toxicity Mediated by Couples

Multigenerational Studies	*Other Reproductive Endpoints*
Mating rate, time to mating (time to pregnancy)	Ovulation rate
Pregnancy rate	Fertilization rate
Delivery rate	Preimplantation loss
Gestation length	Implantation number
Litter size (total and live)	Post implantation loss
Number of live and dead offspring (fetal death rate)	Internal malformations
Offspring gender (sex ratio)	
Birth weight	

Multigenerational Studies	*Other Reproductive Endpoints*
Postnatal weights	
Offspring survival	
External malformations and variations	
Offspring reproduction	

Indices that can be calculated from endpoints of reproductive toxicity in test species

Mating Index

$$\frac{\text{Number of males or females who have mated}}{\text{Number of males or females cohabited}} \times 100$$

Fertility Index

$$\frac{\text{Number of female cohabitees who become pregnant}}{\text{Number of non-pregnant couples cohabited}} \times 100$$

Pregnancy Index

$$\frac{\text{Number of females who give birth to live infants}}{\text{Number of females who have signs of pregnancy}} \times 100$$

Live Birth Index

$$\frac{\text{Number of live infants}}{\text{Number of female offspring}} \times 100$$

Sex Ratio

$$\frac{\text{Number of male infants}}{\text{Number of female infants}}$$

Viability Index

$$\frac{\text{Number of live offspring on day 4 of lactation}}{\text{Number of live offspring}}$$

Weaning Index

$$\frac{\text{Number of live offspring at day 21}}{\text{Number of live offspring born}} \times 100$$

Preweaning Index

$$\frac{\text{Number of offspring weaned}}{\text{Number of live offspring born}} \times 100$$

Mating Rate

Mating rate may be reported for the mated pairs, males only or females only. Direct observation of copulation, observation of copulatory plugs, or observation of sperm in the vaginal fluid can all be used as evidence of mating (vaginal lavage). The number of estrous cycles allowed or required for pregnancy may influence the mating rate. As a result, measurements based on the first estrous cycle after the start of cohabitation should be more discriminating than those based on multiple cycles. Successful impregnation does not always suggest evidence of mating. The length of time it takes each pair to mate after they begin cohabitation could be a useful indicator of impaired reproductive function (time to mating). An increased time between the start of cohabitation and evidence of mating suggests that the female has abnormal estrous cyclicity or that one or both partners have impaired sexual behaviour.

Fertilization Rate

Because the measurement requires necropsy very early in gestation, data on fertilization rate, or the proportion of available ova that were fertilized, is rarely available. The pregnancy rate is the percentage of mated couples who have had at least one pregnancy within a given time frame, with pregnancy determined by the earliest available evidence of fertilization. When the mating opportunity was limited to one mating couple and one estrous cycle, a more meaningful measure of fertility was obtained.

The integrity and timing of gamete and zygote transport are critical for fertilization and embryo survival, and they are highly susceptible to chemical perturbation. Preimplantation loss is a term used to describe the disruption of processes that lead to a lower fertilization rate and more-early embryo loss. To determine the cause of increased preimplantation loss, more research using direct assessments of fertilized ova and early embryos is needed [16]. Preimplantation loss occurs in both untreated and treated rodents, and it contributes to litter size variation.

Uterine and oviduct contractions are important in the transport of spermatozoa from the vaginal canal after mating. The initiation of those contractions in rodents requires sufficient stimulation during mating. As a result, sperm transport and fertilization rate may be affected by poor mating behaviour. The female's gamete transport can be affected by estrogenic compounds. Low doses of exogenous estrogens may hasten ovum transport in female, whereas high doses of estrogens or progestin delay transport and increase the risk of ectopic pregnancies in female.

Mammalian ova are enclosed in different layers, which sperm must pass through before fusing with the ova. Chemicals can obstruct fertilization by obstructing this pathway. Other agents may interfere with sperm fusion with the oolemma, sperm or ovum chromatin transformations into male and female pronuclei, pronuclei fusion, or subsequent cleavage divisions. Carbendazim, a microtubule synthesis inhibitor, is one example of a chemical that can affect meiosis and thus interfere with oocyte maturation and normal zygote formation after sperm-egg fusion [17, 18]. Mutagens such as ethylene oxide can cause harm to the early zygote [19]. Due to the limited sensitivity of rodent fertility measures, a NOAEL, LOAEL, or benchmark dose based on fertility may not accurately reflect the extent of the toxic effect.

Data from additional reproductive endpoints may indicate that an adverse effect could occur at a lower dose level in such cases. In the absence of such information, the exposure margin or uncertainty factor applied to the NOAEL, LOAEL, or benchmark dose may need to be adjusted to account for the additional uncertainty.

The blastocyst and the uterus must both be ready for implantation, and their development must occur at the same time [16]. The uterine endometrium is prepared for implantation by estrogen and progesterone stimulation in a specific order. Treatments that disrupt the internal hormonal environment or inhibit protein synthesis, mitosis, or cell differentiation can prevent implantation and result in the death of the embryo.

Gestation Length

Data on the day of mating (observation of vaginal plug or sperm-positive vaginal lavage) and the day of parturition can be used to calculate gestation length in test animals. Significantly shortened gestation can result in negative pregnancy outcomes such as lower birth weight and offspring survival. Failure of the normal mechanism for parturition may cause significantly longer gestation, which may result in death or impairment of the offspring if dystocia (difficulty in parturition) occurs. Dystocia is a threat to maternal health in both humans and test animals. Although this comparison is complicated by generally faster postnatal growth rates than in utero, comparing offspring weights based on conception age may provide insight.

Litter Size

The number of offspring delivered is measured at or shortly after birth and is referred to as the litter size. Because of dam cannibalism, the number of offspring observed may be less than the actual number delivered unless this observation is made soon after parturition. The number of ova available for fertilization (ovulation rate), fertilization rate, implantation rate, and the proportion of implanted embryos that survive to parturition all influence the size of the litter. Because the number of live and dead offspring in a litter can vary, data on the number of live and dead offspring should be available as well.

Pregnancy status, including pre- and post-implantation losses, can be determined when pregnant animals are necropsied in the middle to late stages of pregnancy. Examining uterus from post parturient females can also reveal post implantation loss. Following the delivery of a litter, post-implantation loss is calculated as (total number of implantation sites minus number of full-term pups)/ number of implantation sites.

Offspring Gender

In mammals, the male determines the gender of the offspring by fertilizing an ovum with Y- or X-chromosome-bearing sperm. As a result, a change in the sex ratio can be caused by a selective impairment in the production, transport, or fertilizing ability of either of these sperm types. Male or female fetuses may be lost selectively if an agent is used. Furthermore, agents that disrupt sexual development may alter the external sexual characteristics of offspring, resulting in apparent effects on sex ratios. These factors are not routinely examined and these factors are the most likely explanations for changes in the sex ratio.

Birth Weight

On the day of delivery, the weight of the infants should be measured. Individual pup data, as well as the litter's total weight (litter weight), are frequently provided. Intrauterine growth rates, litter size, and gestation length all influence birth weight. The normal fetus, the maternal environment, and gender all influence growth rate in utero, with females being smaller than males [20]. Puppies from large litters are typically smaller than pups from smaller litters. Reduced birth weights due to large litter sizes should not be considered an adverse effect unless the increased litter size is due to a treatment and the offspring's ability to survive or develop is harmed as a result. Puppies' weights can be adjusted for litter size using multivariate analyses (*e.g.*, analysis of covariance, multiple regression). When only litter weights are reported, the increased number of offspring and lower individual weights tend to cancel each other. When an acute exposure impairs prenatal or postnatal growth, compensatory growth after dosing cessation may obscure the earlier effect.

Postnatal Weights

Postnatal weights are determined by the individual's birth weight, sex, and normalcy, as well as the litter size, dam lactational ability, and offspring suckling ability. Small or weak offspring may struggle to compete for milk in large litters, resulting in stunted growth. In the absence of contrary evidence, growth retardation or a lower survival rate should be considered negative. In addition, offspring weights in very small litters may appear normal and should be carefully compared to controls.

Offspring Survival

It is influenced by the same factors that influence postnatal weight, though more severe effects are usually required to affect survival. Toxicology of an agent can affect all weight and survival endpoints, either directly on the offspring or indirectly through effects on the dam's ability to support the offspring.

Sexual Behaviour

Sexual behaviour is a complex interaction of neural, endocrine, and reproductive organs that can be disrupted by a variety of toxic agents and pathologic conditions. Environmental agents interfering with sexual behaviour in either sex is a potentially serious in human reproductive. The majority of human data comes from studies on the effects of drugs on sexual behaviour or clinical reports in which exposure-effect associations are unlikely to be found. Data on sexual behaviour is rarely available from studies of human populations exposed to potentially toxic agents in the workplace or in the environment, nor is it routinely obtained in studies of environmental agents with test species.

Most breeding studies do not conduct a direct evaluation of this behaviour. Copulatory plugs or sperm-positive vaginal lavages, on the other hand, are used to demonstrate sexual receptivity and successful mating. These markers, however, do not show whether male performance resulted in adequate female sexual stimulation. Failure of the male to provide adequate stimulation to the female may impair sperm transport in the female rat's genital tract, lowering the chances of successful fertilization [21]. Such a "mating" failure would show up in the calculated fertility index as lower fertility, which could be attributed incorrectly to an effect on the male spermatogenic process or female fertility.

The occurrence of lordosis in rats is a direct indicator of female sexual receptivity. The female rat's sexual receptivity is normally cyclic, with receptivity beginning in the late evening of vaginal pro-estrus. Agents that disrupt normal estrous cyclicity may also result in a lack of or abnormal sexual behaviour, as evidenced by a decrease in the number of females with vaginal plugs or sperm, changes in lordosis behaviour, and a longer time between mating and the start of cohabitation. Latency periods to first mount, mount with intromission, and first ejaculation, number of mounts with intromission to ejaculation, and the postejaculatory interval are among the male measures [22].

For all agents being tested for reproductive toxicity, a direct assessment of sexual behaviour is not required. Agents that have been reported to cause central or peripheral neurotoxicity are possible candidates. Chemicals with or suspected androgenic or estrogenic properties (or antagonistic properties) should also be considered as having the potential to have negative effects on sexual behaviour as well as the reproductive organs.

Table 8.2: Endpoints that are Specific to Male

Male-specific endpoints of reproductive toxicity are	
Organ weights	Testes, epididymis, seminal vesicles, prostate, pituitary
Visual examination and histopathology	Testes, epididymis, seminal vesicles, prostate
Sperm evaluation	Sperm number (count) and quality (morphology, motility)
Sexual behavior	Mounts, intromissions, ejaculations
Hormone levels	LH, FSH, testosterone, estrogen, prolactin
Developmental effects	Testis descent, preputial separation, sperm production, ano-genital distance, str. of ext. genital

Body Weight and Organ Weights

Body weight monitoring during treatment provides an indicator of the animals' overall health, and this information could be useful in interpreting reproductive effects. Weight loss or gain may be due to a variety of factors, including reduced palatability of chemical-containing food or water, treatment-induced anorexia, or systemic toxicity. Male reproductive organs and function have been shown to be unaffected by less severe reductions in adult body weight caused by restricted nutrition [23, 24]. It is not appropriate to dismiss significant alteration of the male reproductive system as secondary to the occurrence of non-reproductive toxicity when a meaningful, biologic relationship between a body weight loss and a significant effect on the male reproductive system is not apparent. In the presence of mild to moderate body weight changes, a change in a reproductive measure that would otherwise be considered adverse should still be considered an adverse male reproductive effect unless additional data provide the needed clarification. It should be noted that an adverse effect on a reproductive endpoint occurred in the presence of severe body weight depression or other severe systemic debilitation, but the effect could have been due to a more generalized toxic effect. Regardless, in that situation, negative effects would have been observed, and a risk assessment should be pursued if sufficient data is available. The testes, epididymis, pituitary gland, seminal vesicles (with coagulating glands), and prostate are among the male reproductive organs for which weights may be useful in determining reproductive risk. Data on organ weights can be presented as absolute or relative weights (*i.e.*, organ weight to body weight ratios). Since the weight of the brain is usually stable after development, it is reported in terms of brain weight [25]. Data on absolute organ weights must be analyzed because a decrease in reproductive organ weight may occur without being related to a decrease in body weight gain. If both body weight and organ weight change in the same direction, the organ weight-to-body weight ratio may not show a significant difference, masking an organ weight effect. Within a test species, normal testis weight varies slightly [26, 27]. Because of the low inter-animal variability, absolute testis weight appears to be a good predictor of gonadal injury. On the other hand damage to the testes can only be detected as a weight change at doses higher than those required to produce significant effects in other gonadal status indicators [28-30]. This inconsistency could be caused by a delay before cell deaths manifest as a weight loss or leydig cell hyperplasia. Blockage of the efferent ducts by cells sloughed from the germinal epithelium or the efferent ducts themselves can result in an increase in testis weight due to fluid accumulation, an effect that could counteract the effect of germinal epithelium depletion on testis weight [31, 32], While testis weight measurements may not reflect all adverse testicular effects or the nature of an effect, a significant increase or decrease in testis weight is indicative of an adverse effect.

Pituitary gland weight can reveal important information about an animal's reproductive status. On the other hand the pituitary contains cell types that regulate a variety of physiologic functions, including some that are unrelated to reproduction. As a result, changes in pituitary weight may not always indicate a problem with reproduction. Gonadotroph-specific histopathologic evaluations may be useful in identifying the affected cell types if weight changes are observed. This information can then be used to determine whether the pituitary effect is linked to reproductive system function and thus has a negative reproductive effect.

The weights of the prostate and seminal vesicles are androgen-dependent and may reflect endocrine or testicular function changes in the animal. In rodents, separating the seminal vesicles from the coagulating gland (dorsal prostate) is difficult. On the other hand seminal vesicle and prostate can be separated and results for these glands can be reported separately or together with or without their secretory fluids. Artefactual weights could result from differential secretory fluid loss prior to weighing. Because the seminal vesicles and prostate may react to an agent differently (endocrine dependency and developmental susceptibility differ), examining the weights separately may yield more information.

Evaluations of Histopathology

Male reproductive risk assessment relies mainly on histopathologic examinations of test animal tissues. The testes, epididymis, prostate, seminal vesicles (often including coagulating glands), and pituitary are all frequently examined organs. Tissues from lower dose exposures are frequently not histologically examined if the high dose had no effect on the controls. Histologic evaluations are particularly useful because they provide- a relatively sensitive indicator of damage, information on toxicity from a variety of protocols, information on site (including target cells) and extent of toxicity with short-term dosing and indicate the potential for recovery with short-term dosing.

Proper fixation and embedding of testicular tissue improves the quality of information presented from histologic analyses of spermatogenesis. A description of the nature and background level of lesions in control tissue, whether preparation-induced or not, can help interpret the nature and extent of lesions observed in tissues obtained from exposed animals when properly prepared tissue is available [33-35]. If the germinal epithelium is severely depleted or degenerating, if multinucleated giant cells are visible, or if sloughed cells are present in the tubule lumen, many histopathologic examinations of the testis will only detect lesions. When less than adequate tissue preparation methods are used, more subtle lesions, such as retained spermatids or missing germ cell types, that can significantly affect the number of sperm released normally into the tubule lumen, may go undetected. Also, familiarity with the detailed morphology of the testis and the kinetics of spermatogenesis of each test species can aid in the detection of less obvious lesions that may accompany lower dose exposures or lesions that occur after a short period of exposure [34]. The technique of "staging" is one of several approaches for qualitative or quantitative assessment of testicular tissue that can aid in the identification of less obvious lesions that may accompany lower-dose exposures.

Histologic evaluation of the epididymis and accessory sex glands is usually limited to the height and possibly integrity of the secretory epithelium. Information on the epididymis' caput, corpus, and cauda segments should be included in the evaluation. Damage to the germinal epithelium or the excurrent ducts is indicated by the presence of debris and sloughed cells in the epididymal lumen. The presence of lesions in the cauda epididymal epithelium, such as sperm granulomas, leucocyte infiltration (inflammation), or the absence of clear cells, should be noted. The morphology of the cell types that produce the gonadotropins and prolactin should be evaluated as part of pituitary examinations.

Data from histopathologic evaluations may provide a relatively sensitive tool for detecting low-dose effects if properly obtained (*i.e.*, proper preparation and analysis of tissue). This method could also reveal the agent's sites and mechanisms of action on that reproductive organ. When humans have similar targets or mechanisms, the foundation for interspecies extrapolation is strengthened. Information can also be obtained, depending on the experimental design that may allow prediction of the eventual extent of injury and degree of recovery in that species and humans [36].

Sperm Analysis

Sperm number, morphology, and motility are all important parameters to consider when evaluating sperm. Data on those parameters allows for a more accurate estimate of the number of "normal" sperm, which is likely to be more insightful than sperm count alone. While other measures such as testicular spermatid count or cauda epididymal weight may reflect effects on sperm development, no substitute measures are adequate to reflect effects on sperm morphology or motility. Human ejaculates may provide similar data without being invasive, improving the ability to validate or detect results observed in research animals. Sperm number or sperm concentration from test species may be derived from ejaculated, epididymal, or testicular samples [37]. Ejaculates can only be obtained readily from rabbits or dogs also can be recovered from the reproductive tracts of mated females of other species [38]. If spermatid counts are available, the ability to detect a decline in testicular sperm production may be improved. On the other hand spermatid counts represent the health of spermatogenic processes within the testes. Only epididymal, vas deferens, or ejaculated samples may be used to assess post testicular effects or toxicity which are expressed as changes in motility, morphology, viability, fragility, and other sperm properties.

The structural characteristics of sperm can be analyzed in cauda epididymal, vas deferens, or ejaculated samples. Abnormalities in the sperm head and flagellum are found after a careful morphologic examination. Sperm head morphology has been a commonly recorded sperm variable in toxicology studies on test species due to the implied association between an agent's mutagenicity and its capacity to trigger abnormal sperm [39]. The common assumption has been that an increase in sperm head malformations is due to germ-cell mutagenicity. However, not all mutagen causes sperm head defects and non-mutagenic chemicals can also change the shape of sperm heads. For example microtubule poisons can increase the incidence of irregular sperm heads by interfering with spermiogenesis, a microtubule-dependent mechanism [40]. Sperm morphology can be altered as a result of cell death-induced degeneration. As a result, the relationship between sperm morphology and mutagenicity is neither responsive nor unique. Sperm morphology profiles in a normal test species (and a strain within a species) are relatively stable and consistent over time. In healthy test species, sperm morphology is one of the least volatile sperm measurements, which can make it more useful in detecting spermatotoxic events [41]. On the other hand, the reproductive effects of different forms of irregular sperm morphology need to be clarified further. The majority of research in laboratory animals and humans suggests that sperm with unusual shapes may not enter the oviduct or engage in fertilization [42, 43].

The biochemical environments in the testes and epididymis are precisely regulated to ensure proper sperm production and maturation, as well as the acquisition of functional characteristics such as progressive motility and fertilization ability. This balance can be disrupted by chemical exposures, resulting in changes in sperm properties such as motility. Chemicals that selectively influence sperm motility and reduce fertility have been reported (*e.g.*, epichlorohydrin). Rat sperm motility has been studied as a reproductive endpoint [44-47] and sperm motility tests are used in some reproductive toxicity tests [48-50]. Vas deferens, cauda epididymal and ejaculated samples can be used to assess motility. Since motility is influenced by a number of experimental variables, such as abstinence interval, sample collection and handling method, elapsed time between sampling and observation, temperature at which the sample is stored and analysed, the extent of sperm dilution, the nature of the dilution medium, and the microscopic chamber used for the observation, standardised methods are needed [51-55]. Sperm motility can be assessed in live samples using phase contrast microscopy, or sperm images can be captured and stored in video or digital format for later analysis, either manually or using computer-assisted semen analysis [56-60]. The percentage of motile and increasingly motile sperm can be measured manually, and the vigour of the sperm motion can be defined using a simple scale. As a result, providing information on a variety of sperm measures as well as reproductive organ histopathology, in addition to fertility, aids the process of determining reproductive risk.

Endpoints that are Specific to Female

The reproductive life cycle of the female may be divided into phases that include fetal, prepubertal, cycling adult, pregnant, lactating, and reproductively senescent. All phases have detailed descriptions available [61]. It is critical to detect negative effects at any of these stages. Traditionally, endpoints have focused on the ability to become pregnant, the outcome of the pregnancy, and the survival and development of the offspring. Although test species can obtain reproductive organ weights and have these organs histologically examined, these measures do not always detect abnormalities in dynamic processes like estrous cyclicity or follicular atresia unless the degradation is severe. Similarly, neither the toxic effects on the onset of puberty nor the long-term effects of exposure on reproductive senescence have been studied. As a result, the amount of data collected on a regular basis to detect toxic effects on the female reproductive system is limited. At dose levels below those that cause reduced fertility or other overt effects on pregnancy or pregnancy outcomes, adverse changes in the nonpregnant female reproductive system have been observed [62-65]. The status of the normal female reproductive system fluctuates in adults, unlike the male reproductive system. The ovarian structures and other reproductive organs change throughout the estrous or menstrual cycle in non-pregnant animals (including humans).

Normal changes accompany the progression of pregnancy, lactation, and the return to cyclicity during or after lactation, though they are not cyclic. These natural fluctuations may have an impact on the evaluation endpoints. As a result, knowing the female's reproductive status at necropsy, including the stage of the estrous cycle, can help with the detection and interpretation of effects with endpoints like uterine weight and ovary and uterus histopathology. With such measures, necropsy of all test animals at the same stage of the estrous cycle can reduce the variance of test results.

Toxicity studies have used a variety of methods to assess the health of the female reproductive system. A comprehensive evaluation of the reproductive process, including identification of target organs and possible elucidation of the mechanisms involved in the agent's effect, can be achieved with the right measures. The central nervous system (particularly the hypothalamus), the pituitary, the ovaries, the reproductive tract, and the secondary sexual organs all play a role in female reproductive function. Other non-gonadotrophic endocrine system components may also influence reproductive system function. Because certain important aspects of female reproductive function (*e.g.*, increased rate of follicular atresia, ovulation failure) are difficult to measure, an assessment of endocrine status may provide needed information that would be unavailable.

The relationships between the various reproductive hormones and the female reproductive organs must be understood in order to understand the significance of effects on reproductive endpoints. Although some effects may be labelled as harmful on a regular basis, all results should be viewed in the context of known biology.

The female reproductive endpoints are presented in a different format than the male reproductive endpoints in order to examine events that are linked and fluctuate with changing endocrine status. For each organ, the organ weight, gross morphology, and histology are all combined. The non-pregnant animal is used to discuss endpoints and endocrine factors for the individual female reproductive organs. Then there's a look at 37 cyclicity measures and how they're interpreted. Then there are considerations for prepubescent, pregnant, lactating, and ageing females.

Table 8.3: Female-Specific Endpoints of Reproductive Toxicity

Organ weights	Ovary, uterus, vagina, pituitary
Visual examination	Ovary, uterus, vagina, pituitary, oviduct, mammary gland and histopathology
Estrous (menstrual)	Vaginal smear cytology cycle normality
Sexual behavior	Lordosis, time to mating, vaginal plugs, or sperm
Hormone levels	LH, FSH, estrogen, progesterone, prolactin
Lactation	Offspring growth, milk quantity and quality
Development	Normality of external genitalia, vaginal opening, vaginal smear cytology, onset of estrous behavior
Senescence	Vaginal smear cytology, ovarian histology

Body Weight, Organ Weight, Organ Morphology, and Histology

Toxicologists are frequently concerned about the effects of changing body weight on reproductive function. Because estrogen and progesterone are known to influence food intake and energy expenditure to a significant extent in females, body weight fluctuates normally with the physiologic state of the animal [66, 67]. The rate of fat deposition and water retention are also influenced [68,69]. Because of the increased serum progesterone level, food consumption increases during pregnancy. A decrease in food intake and body weight in female rats is one of the most sensitive noninvasive indicators of a compound with estrogenic action. Growth retardation caused by extra gonadal hormone effects (*e.g.*, thyroid or growth hormone) can also cause pubertal development to be delayed, as well as acyclicity and infertility. Except in extreme cases, the weights of the reproductive organs are poorly correlated with body weight due to these endocrine-related fluctuations. For the female reproductive system, actual organ weight data rather than organ to body weight ratios should be reported and evaluated.

Chapin investigated the effects of food restriction on female Sprague Dawley rats and Swiss CD-1 mice with body weights of 90 per cent, 80 per cent, and 70 per cent of controls. Female rats were resistant to effects on reproductive function at 80 per cent of control weight, whereas mice had negative effects at 80 per cent of control weight and a marginal effect at 90 per cent. These findings suggest that the female rodent reproductive system responds differently to reduce food intake or body weight reduction depending on the species (and probably the strain).

Ovary

The ovary is responsible for a variety of reproductive functions, including the production and ovulation of oocytes. Estrogen is produced by follicles that are developing, and progesterone is produced by corpora lutea, which are formed after ovulation.

Ovarian Mass

Significant changes in ovarian weight when compared to controls should be taken as a sign of female reproductive toxicity. Although ovarian function changes throughout the estrous cycle, ovarian weight does not change significantly in the normal rat. Still, ovarian weight changes may be linked to oocyte and follicle depletion, persistent polycystic ovaries, inhibition of corpus luteum formation, luteal cyst development, reproductive ageing, and altered hypothalamic-pituitary function. As a result, it's critical to look at ovarian gross morphology and histology to see if changes in those parameters correlate with changes in ovarian weight. However, not all ovarian histologic changes occur at the same time as ovarian weight changes. As a result, the absence of an effect on organ weights does not rule out the need for a histologic examination.

Histopathology

The epithelial capsule and ovarian stroma, as well as the three major compartments of the ovary (*i.e.*, follicular, luteal, and interstitial), may indicate ovarian toxicity. Ovarian histology can detect a variety of pathologic conditions [70,71]. There are methods for determining the number of follicles and their 40 stages of maturation [72]. When a compound depletes the pool of primordial follicles or alters their subsequent development and recruitment during the events leading up to ovulation, these techniques may be useful.

Adverse Effect

Any of the following effects that cause significant changes in the ovaries should be considered harmful:

- Increase or decrease in ovarian weight
- Increased incidence of follicular atresia
- Decreased number of primary follicles
- Decreased number or lifespan of corpora lutea
- Evidence of abnormal folliculogenesis or luteinization, including cystic follicles, luteinized follicles, and failure of ovulation
- Evidence of altered puberty or premature reproductive senescence

Weight of the Uterus

A change in the weight of the uterus could be a sign of toxicity in the female reproductive organs. Inhibitors of steroidogenesis and cyclicity can dramatically reduce uterine weight, making it appear atrophic and small. However, uterine weight varies three to fourfold throughout the estrous cycle, peaking at pro-estrus when the uterus is fluid-filled and distended in response to increased estrogen secretion. In bioassays, this increase in uterine weight has been used to compare the relative potency of estrogenic compounds [73]. Uterine weights taken from cycling animals have a high variance due to the wide fluctuations in weight, and large compound-related effects are required to demonstrate a significant effect unless interpreted relative to that animal's estrous cycle stage. Pesticides like methoxychlor and chlordecone, mycotoxins, polychlorinated biphenyls, alkylphenols, and phytoestrogens have estrogenic activity in varying degrees and have the potential to stimulate the female reproductive tract [74-76]. The number of implantation sites or implantation scars should be counted when pregnant or postpartum animals are examined. Pre- and post-implantation losses can be calculated using this information, as well as corpus luteum counts.

Histopathology

The normal uterus' histologic appearance varies depending on the stage of the estrous cycle and pregnancy. Estrogens have a strong influence on the uterine endometrium. Warren et al. (1967) discovered that progestogens cause hypertrophy and hyperplasia when used for a long time. Endometrial hypoplasia and atrophy, as well as altered vaginal smear cytology, occur when ovarian activity is inhibited and steroid secretion is reduced. Puberty may be delayed or prevented as a result of effects induced during development, resulting in the persistence of infantile genitalia.

Oviducts

In most reproductive toxicity tests, the oviducts are not weighed or histologically examined. Visual and histologic examinations are useful in detecting morphologic abnormalities. It's rare to find descriptions of pathologic effects in the oviducts of animals other than humans. Lack of estrogen stimulation causes hypoplasia of well-formed oviducts and loss of cilia, which is why this condition may not be recognised until after puberty. Prolonged estrogenic stimulation causes hyperplasia of the oviductal epithelium. Agenesis, segmental aplasia, and hypoplasia have all been described as anomalies induced during development. Anatomic anomalies in the oviduct that occur at a rate higher than the control rate should be considered adverse effects. Hypoplasia or hyperplasia of the oviductal epithelium may be considered a side effect, especially if the result is consistent with uterine histology findings.

Vagina and External Genitalia

Vaginal Weight

The changes in vaginal weight should be similar to those in the uterus during the estrous cycle, though the magnitude of the changes should be smaller.

Histopathology

The different stages of the estrous cycle in rodents can be identified by cytologic changes in the vaginal epithelium (vaginal smear). The vaginal smear pattern may be useful in detecting conditions that affect sexual behaviour or delay or prevent fertility. Aplasia, hypoplasia, and hyperplasia of the vaginal epithelial cell lining are some of the other histologic changes that can be seen.

Developmental Effects

Agenesis, hypoplasia, and dysgenesis are developmental defects caused by either hereditary or prenatal exposure to compounds that disturb the endocrine balance. Vaginal hypoplasia may occur in conjunction with external genital hyperplasia and can be triggered by gonadal or adrenal steroid exposure. Malpositioning of the vaginal and urethral ducts in steroid-treated female rodents is normal. These types of developmentally mediated lesions are permanent. Exposure of genotypic females in utero to agents that disrupt reproductive tract development can affect the sex ratio observed at birth. Female rodents that have undergone incomplete sex reversal as a result of such exposures can appear more male-like and have a greater ano-genital gap [77]. The opening of the vaginal orifice provides a basic and useful developmental marker during puberty. Estrogenic or antiestrogenic chemicals may function directly on the vaginal epithelium and change the age at which vaginal patency occurs without affecting puberty.

Pituitary Weight

Changes in pituitary gland weight should be considered as a negative effect. The weight of the pituitary gland rises with age, as well as during pregnancy and lactation. Pituitary weight changes may also occur as a result of chemical stimulation. Increased pituitary weight often precedes tumour formation, particularly when estrogenic compounds are used. Hyperprolactinemia and constant vaginal estrus can accompany increased pituitary size caused by oestrogen therapy. Reduced pituitary weight is less common, but it can be caused by a reduction in estrogenic stimulation [78].

Histopathology

The relative size of cell types in the anterior pituitary has been reported to differ with the stages of the menstrual cycle and during pregnancy in histologic studies with rats and mice. As a result, when analysing histologic findings on the female pituitary, the relationship of morphologic pattern to estrous or menstrual cycle stage or pregnancy status should be taken into account [79]. An adverse effect will be a substantial rise or decrease in pituitary weight. Significant histopathologic damage in the pituitary can be considered an adverse effect, but to be called a reproductive effect, it must be shown to include cells that regulate gonadotropin or prolactin output.

Oocyte Production

Folliculogenesis

Both of the follicles (as well as the resident oocytes) are present in normal females at or shortly after birth. The majorities of these follicles develops atresia and are not fertilized. If the follicle population is reduced, it cannot be replenished, and the female becomes infertile. Oocyte loss causes premature menopause in humans. Crisp has studied the biology and toxicology of ovarian follicles [80]. Lead, arsenic, cadmium, and polyaromatic hydrocarbons have all been linked to the blocking of follicular development in rodents at different stages of their lives [81]. Oocyte toxicity susceptibility varies greatly between species [82]. Environmental factors that influence gonadotropin-mediated ovarian steroidogenesis or follicular maturation may prolong the follicular phase of the estrous or menstrual cycle, resulting in atresia of ovulating follicles. This effect can be caused by both estrogenic and anti-estrogenic agents. Normal follicular maturation is also essential for the proper development and function of the corpus luteum, which is developed after ovulation [83].

Ovulation

Chemicals may cause ovulation to be delayed or prevented by disrupting the luteinizing hormone (LH) ovulatory surge or interfering with the maturing follicle's ability to react to the gonadotropic signal. Compounds that interfere with normal CNS norepinephrine receptor stimulation, such as the pesticides chlordimeform and amitraz and compounds that interfere with norepinephrine synthesis, such as the fungicide thiram [84, 85]. In monkeys and rats, compounds that increase central opioid receptor stimulation often reduce serum LH and inhibit ovulation. Delayed ovulation can affect oocyte viability and result in conceptus trisomy and polyploidy [86-91]. In rats, delayed ovulation caused by the pesticide chlordimeform has been shown to affect foetal development and pregnancy outcome.

Corpus luteum

The corpus luteum is formed when a follicle ruptures and secretes progesterone, which is essential in the estrous or menstrual cycle. In most mammalian species, including humans, luteal progesterone is also required for the maintenance of early pregnancy [92]. As a result, normal corpora lutea formation and maintenance are critical for normal reproductive function. These structures are not tested in routine examination, with the exception of histopathologic tests that can only determine their presence or absence. More research is required to decide how important it is to have endpoints that look at direct effects.

The sequence of events in the estrous cycle can be a good predictor of the non-pregnant female's reproductive neuroendocrine and ovarian function. It can also be used to monitor the status of mated females by interpreting hormonal, histologic, and morphologic measurements in relation to the stage of the cycle. The normalcy of the estrous cycle in the rat and mouse can be determined by studying changes in vaginal smear cytology. Vaginal smear cytology should be tested regularly for at least three natural estrous cycles prior to treatment, after treatment begins, and before necropsy in cycling females to be most useful [93-95]. Practical testing restrictions could restrict the analysis to the time leading up to mating or necropsy. Data from daily vaginal smears in rodents can be used to determine cycle length, occurrence or persistence of estrus, period or persistence of diestrus, frequency of spontaneous pseudopregnancy, separating pregnancy from pseudopregnancy (based on the number of days the smear remains leukocytic), and distinguishing pregnancy from pseudopregnancy (based on the number of days the smear remains leukocytic). It is useful further to detect the presence of sperm in the vagina as an indication of mating.

Persistent diestrus means a temporary or permanent stop in follicular growth and ovulation, as well as infertility. Agents (*e.g.*, polyaromatic hydrocarbons) that interfere with follicular production or deplete the pool of primordial follicles or agents such as atrazine that disrupt gonadotropin support of the ovary can cause prolonged vaginal diestrus, or anestrus. Another altered endocrine state reflected by chronic diestrus is pseudo-pregnancy. Following single or multiple doses of atrazine, rats have been shown to develop a pseudo-pregnant disorde. Anestrous females' ovaries are atrophic, with few primary follicles and a uterus that isn't stimulated [96,97]. Estradiol and progesterone levels in the blood are abnormally low.

Mammary Gland and Lactation

Because of the sequential effects of a variety of gonadal and extragonadal hormones, the mammary glands of normal adults shift significantly during the time around parturition. The suckling stimulation and the release of oxytocin from the posterior pituitary are needed for milk letdown. As a result, mammary tissue's growth and function are highly reliant on endocrine signals. Toxic agents may affect mammary gland size, milk development and release, and histology, and many exogenous chemicals and drugs are transferred into milk [98-102]. Reduced young growth may be induced by a lack of milk supply, palatability, or consistency, ingestion of a toxic agent secreted into the milk, or other factors unrelated to lactational ability (*e.g.*, deficient suckling ability or deficient maternal behavior). Adult mammary gland morphology and tumour capacity may be altered by perinatal exposure to steroid hormones and other chemicals. Milk may contain lipophilic agents at concentrations equal to or higher than those present in the dam's blood or organs due to the propensity for lipids to be mobilised from adipose tissue and secreted into milk by lactating females. As a result, suckling offspring can be exposed to high concentrations of such agents. Tucker talks about how to measure mammary tissue growth, nucleic acid content, milk quality, and milk composition in rodents [100]. The mammary glands can only be dissected and measured with difficulty during lactation. The RNA content of mammary glands can be used to determine lactational potential. Measurement of litter weights of milk-deprived pups before and after nursing will provide more direct estimates of milk production. At necropsy, milk from the stomachs of pups handled similarly may also be measured. At necropsy, entire mounts of the mammary gland that have been cleared and stained can be prepared for histologic inspection. Following toxicant administration, the DNA, RNA, and lipid content of the mammary gland, as well as the composition of the milk, were assessed as measures of toxicity to this target organ. Significant decreases in milk production or detrimental effects on milk quality, whether directly assessed or expressed in impaired young growth, should be considered adverse reproductive effects.

Reproductive Senescence

The daily ovarian cycles and associated natural cyclical changes in the uterine and vaginal epithelium that are typical of the young-adult female rat are lost with age. Although the mechanisms underlying this loss of cycling are unknown, age-related changes in the hypothalamic-pituitary regulation of ovulation do occur [103-105]. Treatment with estrogens during adulthood may accelerate the age-related loss of ovarian function, so cumulative exposure to oestrogen secreted by the ovary may play a role [106]. The degradation of oocytes, on the other hand, tends to be the primary cause of ovarian cycling loss in humans [107]. Prenatal or postnatal hormone or estrogenic pesticide treatment of females may also result in ovulation problems and sterility [108]. These findings suggest that changes in ovarian function may not be apparent right away after care, but that they may become apparent during puberty or affect the age at which reproductive senescence occurs.

Effect on Puberty

The age at vaginal opening is the most frequently measured marker of puberty in female rats and mice. This occurs as a result of a rise in estradiol levels in the blood. Females' ages and weights at the first cornified (estrous) vaginal smear, the first diestrous smear, and the beginning of vaginal cycles have also been used as endpoints for puberty onset. Preputial separation or the presence of sperm in transmitted urine or ejaculates in males may be used as puberty indicators. Body weight at puberty can be used to distinguish between puberty delays that are linked to general developmental delays.

Exogenous agents can speed up or slow down puberty, and both types of effects can be harmful [109-112]. Accelerated vaginal opening, for example, has been linked to a delay in the onset of cyclicity, infertility, and accelerated reproductive ageing [108]. In rodents, pubertal growth is normally delayed due to hypothalamic-pituitary axis maturation or inhibition of function. When puberty is delayed by a week or more in rodents, negative reproductive outcomes have been identified, but the biologic significance of a day or two in these measures is uncertain [113].

In vitro Tests of Reproductive Function

In vitro experiments to quantify or detect chemically induced changes in various aspects of both male and female reproductive systems are available and in progress [95]. In vitro fertilisation with isolated gametes, whole organ perfusion (*e.g.*, testis, ovary), culture of isolated cells from reproductive organs (*e.g.*, Leydig cells, Sertoli cells, granulosa cells, oviductal or epididymal epithelium), co-culture of many populations of isolated cells, ovaries, quarter testes, seminiferous tubule segments, and various receptor binding assays on reproductive cells. Penetration of sperm by viscous medium, in vitro capacitation and fertilisation assays and assessment of sperm nuclear integrity are all tests of sperm properties and function that have been used in reproductive toxicology [114-117]. Sperm penetration of cervical mucus, ability of sperm to undergo an acrosome reaction, and ability to penetrate zona pellucida-free hamster oocytes or attach to human hemi-zona pellucidae are all examples of human sperm function testing [118, 119].

The diagnostic information obtained from these tests can aid in identifying potential reproductive system effects. However, since each test ignores critical components of the intact animal system, it is unable to predict exposure levels that would cause toxicity in intact animals on its own. Although it would be ideal to replace whole animal testing with in vitro studies to the extent practicable, in vitro tests are currently used to screen for toxicity and study mechanisms of action and metabolism [120].

REFERENCES

1. Goldman, J.M., Cooper, R.L., Edwards, T.L., Rehnberg, G.L., McElroy, W.K., Hein, J.F. (1991) Suppression of the luteinizing hormone surge by chlordimeform in ovariectomized, steroid-primed female rats. Pharmacol. Toxicol. 68:131-136.

2. U.S. Environmental Protection Agency. (1982) Reproductive and Fertility Effects. Pesticide Assessment Guidelines, Subdivision F. Hazard Evaluation: Human and Domestic Animals. Office of Pesticides and Toxic Substances, Washington, D.C. EPA-540/9-82-025.

3. U.S. Environmental Protection Agency. (1985b) Toxic Substances Control Act Test Guidelines: Final Rules. Federal Register 50 (188):39426-39436.

4. U.S. Environmental Protection Agency. (1996a) Health Effects Test Guidelines OPPTS 870.3800: Reproduction and Fertility Effects (Draft). Federal Register 61(43):8282-8283.

5. Galbraith, W.M., Voytek, P., Ryon, M.S. (1983) Assessment of risks to human reproduction and development of the human conceptus from exposure to environmental substances. In: Christian, M.S., Galbraith, W.M., Voytek, P., Mehlman, M.A. Advances in Modern Environmental Toxicology. Princeton Scientific Publ., Princeton. pp. 41-153.

6. Organization for Economic Cooperation and Development. (1983) First addendum to OECD guideline 415 for testing of chemicals, "One-Generation Rreproduction Toxicity."OECD, Paris, pp. 1-8.
7. Francis, E.Z., Kimmel, G.L. (1988) Proceedings of the workshop on one- vs two-generation reproductive effects studies. J. Am. Coll. Toxicol. 7:911-925.
8. Scala, R.A., Bevan, C., Beyer, B.K. (1992) An abbreviated repeat dose and reproductive/developmental toxicity test for high production volume chemicals. Regul. Toxicol. Pharmacol. 16:73-80.
9. Tanaka, S., Kawashima, K., Naito, K., Usami, M., Nakadate, M., Imaida, K., Takahashi, M., Hayashi, Y., Kurokawa, Y., Tobe, M. (1992) Combined repeat dose and reproductive/developmental toxicity screening test (OECD): familiarization using cyclophosphamide. Fundam. Appl. Toxicol. 18:89-95.
10. Organization for Economic Cooperation and Development. (1993a) Draft guidelines for testing chemicals: combined repeated dose toxicity study with the reproduction/developmental toxicity screening test. #422. OECD, Paris.
11. International Conference on Harmonization of Technical Requirements of Pharmaceuticals for Human Use. (1994) ICH harmonized tripartite guideline, Detection of Toxicity to Reproduction for Medicinal Products. Federal Register 59(1831):48746-48752.
12. Manson, J.M. (1994) Testing of pharmaceutical agents for reproductive toxicity. In: Kimmel, C.A., Buelke-Sam, J. Developmental Toxicology. Raven Press, New York. p. 379.
13. Harris, M.W., Chapin, R.E., Lockhart, A.C., Jokinen, M.P., Allen, J.D., Haskins, E.A. (1992) Assessment of a shortterm reproductive and developmental toxicity screen. Fundam. Appl. Toxicol. 19:186-196.
14. Generoso, W.M., Piegorsch, W.W. (1993) Dominant lethal tests in male and female mice. In: Chapin, R.E., Heindel, J.J. Methods in Toxicology: Male Reproductive Toxicology. Academic Press, San Diego. pp. 124-139.
15. U.S. Environmental Protection Agency. (1991) Guidelines for Developmental Toxicity Risk Assessment. Federal Register 56(234):63798-63826.
16. Cummings, A.M., Perreault, S.D. (1990) Methoxychlor accelerates embryo transport through the rat reproductive tract. Toxicol. Appl. Pharmacol. 102:110-116.
17. Perreault, S.D., Jeffay, S., Poss, P., Laskey, J.W. (1992) Use of the fungicide carbendazim as a model compound to determine the impact of acute chemical exposure during oocyte maturation and fertilization on pregnancy outcome in the hamster. Toxicol. Appl. Pharmacol. 114:225-231.
18. Zuelke, K.A., Perreault, S.D. (1995) Carbendazim (MBC) disrupts oocyte spindle function and induces aneuploidy in hamsters exposed during fertilization (meiosis II). Mol. Reprod. Dev. 42:200-209.

19. Generoso, W.M., Rutledge, J.C., Cain, K.T., Hughes, L.A., Braden, P.W. (1987) Exposure of female mice to ethylene oxide within hours after mating leads to fetal malformation and death. Mutat. Res. 176:269-274.

20. Tyl,u R.W. (1987) Developmental toxicity in toxicologic research and testing. In: Ballantyne, B. Perspectives in Basic and Applied Toxicology. John Wright, Bristol. pp. 203-208.

21. Adler, N.T., Toner, J.P. (1986) The effect of copulatory behavior on sperm transport and fertility in rats. In: Komisaruk, B.R., Siegel, H.I., Chang, M.F., Feder, H.H. Reproduction: Behavioral and Neuroendocrine Perspective. New York Academy of Science, New York. pp. 21-32.

22. Beach, F.A. (1979) Animal models for human sexuality. In: Ciba Foundation Symposium No. 62, Sex, Hormones and Behavior. Elsevier-North Holland, London. pp. 113-143.

23. Chapin, R.E., Gulati, D.K., Barnes, L.H., Teague, J.L. (1993a) The effects of feed restriction on reproductive function in Sprague-Dawley rats. Fundam. Appl. Toxicol. 20:23-29.

24. Chapin, R.E., Gulati, D.K., Fail, P.A., Hope, E., Russell, S.R., Heindel, J.J., George, J.D., Grizzle, T.B., Teague, J.L. (1993b) The effects of feed restriction on reproductive function in Swiss CD-1 mice. Fundam. Appl. Toxicol. 20:15-22.

25. Stevens, K.R., Gallo, M.A. (1989) Practical considerations in the conduct of chronic toxicity studies. In: Hayes, A.W. Principles and Methods of Toxicology. Raven Press, New York. pp. 237-250.

26. Schwetz, B.A., Rao, K.S., Park, C.N. (1980) Insensitivity of tests for reproductive problems. J. Environ. Pathol. Toxicol. 3:81-98.

27. Blazak, W.F., Ernst, T.L., Stewart, B.E. (1985) Potential indicators of reproductive toxicity, testicular sperm production and epididymal sperm number, transit time and motility in Fischer 344 rats. Fundam. Appl. Toxicol. 5:1097-1103.

28. Berndtson, W.E. (1977) Methods for quantifying mammalian spermatogenesis: a review. J. Anim. Sci. 44:818-833.

29. Foote, R.H., Schermerhorn, E.C., Simkin, M.E. (1986) Measurement of semen quality, fertility, and reproductive hormones to assess dibromochloropropane (DBCP) effects in live rabbits. Fundam. Appl. Toxicol. 6:628-637.

30. Ku, W.W., Chapin, R.E., Wine, R.N., Gladen, B.C. (1993) Testicular toxicity of boric acid (BA): relationship of dose to lesion development and recovery in the F344 rat. Reprod. Toxicol. 7:305-319.

31. Hess, R.A., Moore, B.J., Forrer, J., Linder, R.E., Abuel-Atta, A.A. (1991) The fungicide Benomyl (methyl 1(butylcarbamoyl)-2-benzimidazolecarbamate) causes testicular dysfunction by inducing the sloughing of germ cells and occlusion of efferent ductules. Fundam. Appl. Toxicol. 17:733-745.

32. Nakai, M., Moore, B.J., Hess, R.A. (1993) Epithelial reorganization and irregular growth following carbendazim induced injury of the efferent ductules of the rat testis. Anat. Rec. 235:51-60.

33. Chapin, R.E. (1988) Morphologic evaluation of seminiferous epithelium of the testis. In: Lamb, J.C., Foster, P.M.D. Physiology and Toxicology of Male Reproduction. Academic Press, New York. pp. 155-177.

34. Russell, L.D., Ettlin, R., Sinha Hikim, A.P., Clegg, E.D. (1990) Histological and Histopathological Evaluation of the Testis. Cache River Press, Clearwater, FL.

35. Hess, R.A., Moore, B.J. (1993) Histological methods for evaluation of the testis. In: Chapin, R.E., Heindel, J.J. Methods in Toxicology: Male Reproductive Toxicology. Academic Press, San Diego. pp. 52-85.

36. Russell, L.D. (1983) Normal testicular structure and methods of evaluation under experimental and disruptive conditions. In: Clarkson, T.W., Nordberg, G.F., Sager, P.R. Reproductive and Developmental Toxicity of Metals. Plenum Publishing Co., New York. pp. 227-252.

37. Seed, J., Chapin, R.E., Clegg, E.D., Darney, S.P., Dostal, L., Foote, R.H., Hurtt, M.E., Klinefelter, G.R., Makris, S.L., Schrader, S., Seyler, D., Sprando, R., Treinen, K.A., Veeranachaneni, R., Wise, L.D. (1996) Methods for assessing sperm motility, morphology, and counts in the rat, rabbit and dog: a consensus report. Reprod. Toxicol. 10:237-244.

38. Zenick, H., Blackburn, K., Hope, E., Baldwin, D.J. (1984) Evaluating male reproductive toxicity in rodents: a new animal model. Teratogenesis Carcinog. Mutagen. 4:109-128.

39. Wyrobek, A.J., Gordon, L.A., Burkhart, J.G., Francis, M.W., Kapp, R.W., Jr., Letz, G., Malling, H., V, Topham, J.C., Whorton, D.M. (1983b) An evaluation of human sperm as indicators of chemically induced alterations of spermatogenic function. Mutat. Res. 115:73-148.

40. Russell, L.D., Malone, J.P., McCurdy, D.S. (1981) Effect of microtubule disrupting agents, colchicine and vinblastine, on seminiferous tubule structure in the rat. Tissue Cell 13:349-367.

41. Zenick, H., Clegg, E.D., Perreault, S.D., Klinefelter, G.R., Gray, L.E. (1994) Assessment of male reproductive toxicity: a risk assessment approach. In: Hayes, A.W. Principles and Methods of Toxicology. Raven Press, New York. pp. 937-988.

42. Nestor, A., Handel, M.A. (1984) The transport of morphologically abnormal sperm in the female reproductive tract of mice. Gamete Res. 10:119-125.

43. Redi, C.A., Garagna, S., Pellicciari, C., Manfredi-Romanini, M.G., Capanna, E., Winking, H., Gropp, A. (1984) Spermatozoa of chromosomally heterozygous mice and their fate in male and female genital tracts. Gamete Res. 9:273-286.

44. Morrissey, R.E., Lamb, J.C., Schwetz, B.A., Teague, J.L., Morris, R.W. (1988a) Association of sperm, vaginal cytology, and reproductive organ weight data with results of continuous breeding reproduction studies in Swiss (CD-1) mice. Fundam. Appl. Toxicol. 11:359-371.

45. Morrissey, R.E., Schwetz, B.A., Lamb, J.C., Ross, M.D., Teague, J.L., Morris, R.W. (1988b) Evaluation of rodent sperm, vaginal cytology, and reproductive organ

weight data from National Toxicology Program 13-week studies. Fundam. Appl. Toxicol. 11:343-358.

46. Toth, G.P., Zenick, H., Smith, M.K. (1989b) Effects of epichlorohydrin on male and female reproduction in LongEvans rats. Fundam. Appl. Toxicol. 13:16-25.
47. Toth, G.P., Stober, J.A., Zenick, H., Read, E.J., Christ, S.A., Smith, M.K. (1991b) Correlation of sperm motion parameters with fertility in rats treated subchronically with epichlorohydrin. J. Androl. 12:54-61.
48. Gray, L.E., Ostby, J., Sigmon, R., Ferrell, J., Linder, R., Cooper, R., Goldman, J., Laskey, J. (1988). The development of a protocol to assess reproductive effects of toxicants in the rat. Reprod. Toxicol. 2:281-287.
49. Morrissey, R.E., Lamb, J.C., Morris, R.W., Chapin, R.E., Gulati, D.K., Heindel, J.J. (1989) Results and evaluations of 48 continuous breeding reproduction studies conducted in mice. Fundam. Appl. Toxicol. 13:747-777.
50. U.S. Environmental Protection Agency. (1996b) Proposed Guidelines for Carcinogen Risk Assessment. Federal Register 61(79):17960-18011.
51. Slott, V.L., Jeffay, S.C., Suarez, J.D., Barbee, R.R., Perreault, S.D. (1995) Synchronous assessment of sperm motility and fertilizing ability in the hamster following treatment with alpha-chlorohydrin. J. Androl. 16:523-535.
52. Toth, G.P., Stober, J.A., George, E.L., Read, E.J., Smith, M.K. (1991a) Sources of variation in the computer-assisted motion analysis of rat epididymal sperm. Reprod. Toxicol. 5:487-495.
53. Chapin, R.E., Filler, R.S., Gulati, D., Heindel, J.J., Katz, D.F., Mebus, C.A., Obasaju, F., Perreault, S.D., Russell, S.R., Schrader, S., Slott, V., Sokol, R.Z., Toth, G. (1992) Methods for assessing rat sperm motility. Reprod. Toxicol. 6:267273.
54. Schrader, S.M., Chapin, R.E., Clegg, E.D., Davis, R.O., Fourcroy, J.L., Katz, D.F., Rothmann, S.A., Toth, G., Turner, T.W., Zinaman, M. (1992) Laboratory methods for assessing human semen in epidemiologic studies: a consensus report. Reprod. Toxicol. 6:275-279.
55. Weir, P.J., Rumberger, D. (1995) Isolation of rat sperm from the vas deferens for sperm motion analysis. Reprod. Toxicol. 9:327-330.
56. Linder, R.E., Hess, R.A., Strader, L.F. (1986) Testicular toxicity and infertility in male rats treated with l,3dinitrobenzene. J. Toxicol. Environ. Health 19:477-489.
57. Boyers, S.P., Davis, R.O., Katz, D.F. (1989) Automated semen analysis. Curr. Probl. Obstet. Gynecol. Fertil. 12:173200.
58. Toth, G.P., Stober, J.A., Read, E.J., Zenick, H., Smith, M.K. (1989a) The automated analysis of rat sperm motility following subchronic epichlorohydrin administration: methodologic and statistical considerations. J. Androl. 10:401415.
59. Yeung, C.H., Oberlander, G., Cooper, T.G. (1992) Characterization of the motility of maturing rat spermatozoa by computer-aided objective measurement. J. Reprod. Fertil. 96:427-441.

60. Slott, V.L., Perreault, S.D. (1993) Computer-assisted sperm analysis of rodent epididymal sperm motility using the Hamilton-Thorne motility analyzer. In: Chapin, R.E., Heindel, J.J. Methods in Toxicology: Male Reproductive Toxicology. Academic Press, San Diego. pp. 319-333.

61. Knobil, E., Neill, J.D., Greenwald, G.S., Markert, C.L., Pfaff, D.W. (1994) The Physiology of Reproduction. Raven Press, New York.

62. Le Vier, R.R., Jankowiak, M.E. (1972) The hormonal and antifertility activity of 2,6-cis-diphenylhexamethylcyclotetrasiloxane in the female rat. Biol. Reprod. 7:260-266.

63. Barsotti, D.A., Abrahamson, L.J., Allen, J.R. (1979) Hormonal alterations in female rhesus monkeys fed a diet containing 2,3,7,8-TCDD. Bull. Environ. Contam. Toxicol. 21:463-469.

64. Sonawane, B.R., Yaffe, S.J. (1983) Delayed effects of drug exposure during pregnancy: reproductive function. Biol. Res. Pregnancy 4:48-55.

65. Cummings, A.M., Gray, L.E. (1987) Methoxychlor affects the decidual cell response of the uterus but not other progestational parameters in female rats. Toxicol. Appl. Pharmacol. 90:330-336.

66. Wang, G.H. (1923) The relation between the "spontaneous" activity and the oestrous cycle in the white rat. Comp. Psychol. Monographs 2:1-27.

67. Wade, G.N. (1972) Gonadal hormones and behavioral regulation of body weight. Physiol. Behav. 8:523-534.

68. Galletti, F., Klopper, A. (1964) The effect of progesterone on the quantity and distribution of body fat in the female rat. Acta Endocrinol. 46:379-386.

69. Hervey, E., Hervey, G.R. (1967) The effects of progesterone on body weight and composition in the rat. J. Endocrinol. 37:361-384.

70. Kurman, R., Norris, H.J. (1978) Germ cell tumors of the ovary. Pathol. Annu. 13:291.

71. Langley, F.A., Fox, H. (1987) Ovarian tumors. Classification, histogenesis, etiology. In: Fox, H. Haines and Taylor's Obstetrical and Gynaecologic Pathology. Churchill Livingstone, Edinburgh. pp. 542-555.

72. Plowchalk, D.R., Smith, B.J., Mattison, D.R. (1993) Assessment of toxicity to the ovary using follicle quantitation and morphometrics. In: Heindel, J.J., Chapin, R.E. Methods in Toxicology: Female Reproductive Toxicology. Academic Press, San Diego. pp. 57-68.

73. Kupfer, D. (1987) Critical evaluation of methods for detection and assessment of estrogenic compounds in mammals: strengths and limitations for application to risk assessment. Reprod. Toxicol. 2:147-153.

74. Barlow, S.M., Sullivan, F.M. (1982) Reproductive Hazards of Industrial Chemicals. Academic Press, London.

75. Bulger, W.H., Kupfer, D. (1985) Estrogenic activity of pesticides and other xenobiotics on the uterus and male reproductive tract. In: Thomas, J.A., Korach, K.S., McLachlan, J.A. Endocrine Toxicology. Raven Press, New York. pp. 1-33.

76. Hughes, C.L. (1988) Phytochemical mimicry of reproductive hormones and modulation of herbivore fertility by phytoestrogens. Environ Health Perspect. 78:171-175.

77. Gray, L.E., Ostby, J.S. (1995) In utero 2,3,7,8-tetrachlorodibenzo-p-dioxin (TCDD) alters reproductive morphology and function in female rat offspring. Toxicol. Appl. Pharmacol. 133:285-294.

78. Cooper, R.L., Chadwick, R.W., Rehnberg, G.L., Goldman, J.M., Booth, K.C., Hein, J.F., McElroy, W.K. (1989) Effect of lindane on hormonal control of reproductive function in the female rat. Toxicol. Appl. Pharmacol. 99:384-394.

79. Holmes, R.L., Ball, J.N. (1974) The Pituitary Gland: A Comparative Account. Cambridge University Press, Cambridge.

80. Crisp, T.M. (1992) Organization of the ovarian follicle and events in its biology: oogenesis, ovulation or atresia. Mutat. Res. 296:89-106.

81. Mattison, D.R., Thomford, P.J. (1989) The mechanisms of action of reproductive toxicants. Toxicol. Pathol. 17:364376.

82. Mattison, D.R., Thorgeirsson, S.S. (1978) Gonadal aryl hydrocarbon hydroxylase in rats and mice. Cancer Res. 38:1368-1373.

83. McNatty, K.P. (1979) Follicular determinants of corpus luteum function in the human ovary. Adv. Exp. Med. Biol. 112:465-481.

84. Goldman, J.M., Cooper, R.L., Laws, S.C., Rehnberg, G.L., Edwards, T.L., McElroy, W.K., Hein, J.F. (1990) Chlordimeform-induced alterations in endocrine regulation within the male rat reproductive system. Toxicol. Appl. Pharmacol. 104:25-35.

85. Goldman, J.M., Cooper, R.L., Edwards, T.L., Rehnberg, G.L., McElroy, W.K., Hein, J.F. (1991) Suppression of the luteinizing hormone surge by chlordimeform in ovariectomized, steroid-primed female rats. Pharmacol. Toxicol. 68:131-136.

86. Pang, C.N., Zimmerman, E., Sawyer, C.H. (1977) Morphine inhibition of preovulatory surges of plasma luteinizing hormone and follicle stimulating hormone in the rat. Endocrinology 101:1726-1732.

87. Smith, C.G. (1983) Reproductive toxicity: hypothalamic-pituitary mechanisms. Am. J. Ind. Med. 4:107-112

88. Fugo, N.W., Butcher, R.L. (1966) Overripeness and the mammalian ova. I. Overripeness and early embryonic development. Fertil. Steril. 17:804-814.

89. Butcher, R.L., Fugo, N.W. (1967) Overripeness and the mammalian ova. II. Delayed ovulation and chromosome anomalies. Fertil. Steril. 18:297-302.

90. Butcher, R.L., Blue, J.D., Fugo, N.W. (1969) Overripeness and the mammalian ova. III. Fetal development at midgestation and at term. Fertil. Steril. 20:223-231.

91. Butcher, R.L., Collins, W.E., Fugo, N.W. (1975) Altered secretion of gonadotropins and steroids resulting from delayed ovulation in the rat. Endocrinology 96:576-586.

92. Csapo, A.I., Pulkkinen, M. (1978) Indispensability of the human corpus luteum in the maintenance of early pregnancy: lutectomy evidence. Obstet. Gynecol. Surv. 33:69.

93. Long, J.A., Evans, H.M. (1922). The oestrous cycle in the rat and its associated phenomena. Mem. Univ. Calif. 6:1111.

94. Cooper, R.L., Goldman, J.M., Vandenbergh, J.G. (1993) Monitoring of the estrous cycle in the laboratory rodent by vaginal lavage. In: Heindel, J.J., Chapin, R.E. Methods in Toxicology: Female Reproductive Toxicology. Academic Press, San Diego. pp. 45-56.

95. Kimmel, G.L., Clegg, E.D., Crisp, T.M. (1995) Reproductive toxicity testing: a risk assessment perspective. In: Witorsch, R.J. Reproductive Toxicology. Raven Press, New York. pp. 75-98.

96. Mattison, D.R., Nightingale, M.R. (1980) The biochemical and genetic characteristics of murine ovarian aryl hydrocarbon (benzo(a)pyrene) hydroxylase activity and its relationship to primary oocyte destruction by polycyclic aromatic hydrocarbons. Toxicol. Appl. Pharmacol. 56:399-408.

97. Huang, H.H., Meites, J. (1975) Reproductive capacity of aging female rats. Neuroendocrinology 17:289-295.

98. Wolff, M.S. (1993) Lactation. In: Paul, M. Occupational and Environmental Reproductive Hazards. Williams and Wilkins, Baltimore. pp. 60-75.

99. Imagawa, W., Yang, J., Guzman, R., Nandi, S. (1994) Control of mammary gland development. In: Knobil, E., O'Neill, J.D. The Physiology of Reproduction. Raven Press, New York. pp. 1033-1063.

100. Tucker, H.A. (1994) Lactation and its hormonal control. In: Knobil, E., O'Neill, J.D. The Physiology of Reproduction. Raven Press, New York. pp. 1065-1098.

101. American Academy of Pediatrics Committee on Drugs. (1994) The transfer of drugs and other chemicals into human milk. Pediatrics 93:137-150.

102. Oskarsson, A., Hallen, I.P., Sundberg, J. (1995) Exposure to toxic elements via breast milk. Analyst 120:765-770.

103. Cooper, R.L., Walker, R.F. (1979) Potential therapeutic consequences of age-dependent changes in brain physiology. Interdis. Topics Gerontol. 15:54-76.

104. Cooper, R.L., Conn, P.M., Walker, R.F. (1980) Characterization of the LH surge in middle-aged female rats. Biol. Reprod. 23:611-615.

105. Finch, C.E., Felicio, L.S., Mobbs, C.V. (1984) Ovarian and steroidal influences on neuroendocrine aging processes in female rodents. Endocrinol. Rev. 5:467-497.

106. Brawer, J.R., Finch, C.E. (1983) Normal and experimentally altered aging processes in the rodent hypothalamus and pituitary. In: Walker, R.F., Cooper,

R.L. Experimental and Clinical Interventions in Aging. Marcel Dekker, New York. pp. 45-65.

107. Mattison, D.R. (1985) Clinical manifestations of ovarian toxicity. In: Dixon, R.L. Reproductive Toxicology. Raven Press, New York. pp. 109-130.

108. Gorski, R.A. (1979) The neuroendocrinology of reproduction: an overview. Biol. Reprod. 20:111-127.

109. Gray, L.E., Ostby, J., Ferrell, J., Rehnberg, G., Linder, R., Cooper, R., Goldman, J., Slott, V., Laskey, J. (1989) A doseresponse analysis of methoxychlor-induced alterations of reproductive development and function in the rat. Fundam. Appl. Toxicol. 12:92-108.

110. Gray, L.E., Kelce, W.R., Monosson, E., Ostby, J.S., Birnbaum, L.S. (1995) Exposure to TCDD during development permanently alters reproductive function in male Long Evans rats and hamsters: reduced ejaculated and epididymal sperm numbers and sex accessory gland weights in offspring with normal androgenic status. Toxicol. Appl. Pharmacol. 131:108-118.

111. Gray, L.E., Ferrell, J.M., Ostby, J.S. (1985) Alteration of behavioral sex differentiation by exposure to estrogenic compounds during a critical neonatal period: effects of zearalenone, methoxychlor, and estradiol in hamster. Toxicol. Appl. Pharmacol. 80:127-136.

112. Kelce, W.R., Stone, C.R., Laws, S.C., Gray, L.E., Kemppainen, J.A., Wilson, E.M. (1995) Persistent DDT metabolite p,p'-DDE is a potent androgen receptor antagonist. Nature 375:581-585.

113. Gray, L.E. (1991) Delayed effects on reproduction following exposure to toxic chemicals during critical periods of development. In: Cooper, R.L., Goldman, J.M., Harbin, T.J. Aging and Environmental Toxicology: Biological and Behavioral Perspectives. Johns Hopkins University Press, Baltimore. pp. 183-210.

114. Holloway, A.J., Moore, H.D.M., Foster, P.M.D. (1990a) The use of in vitro fertilization to detect reductions in the fertility of male rats exposed to 1,3-dinitrobenzene. Fundam. Appl. Toxicol. 14:113-122.

115. Holloway, A.J., Moore, H.D.M., Foster, P.M.D. (1990b) The use of rat in vitro fertilization to detect reductions in the fertility of spermatozoa from males exposed to ethylene glycol monomethyl ether. Reprod. Toxicol. 4:21-27.

116. Perreault, S.D., Jeffay, S.C. (1993) Strategies and methods for the functional evaluation of oocytes and zygotes. In: Heindel, J.J., Chapin, R.E. Methods in Toxicology: Female Reproductive Toxicology. Academic Press, San Diego. pp. 92-109.

117. Darney, S.P. (1991) In vitro assessment of gamete integrity. In: Goldberg, A.M. In Vitro Toxicology: Mechanisms and New Technology. Mary Ann Liebert, Inc., New York. pp. 63-75.

118. Franken, D.R., Burkman, L.J., Coddington, C.C., Oehninger, S., Hodgen, G.D. (1990) Human hemizona attachment assay. In: Acosta, A.A., Swanson, R.J.,

Ackerman, S.B., Kruger, T.F., VanZyl, J.A., Menkveld, R. Human Spermatozoa in Assisted Reproduction. Williams and Wilkins, Baltimore. pp. 355-371.

119. Liu, D.Y., Baker, H.W.G. (1992) Tests of human sperm function and fertilization in vitro. Fertil. Steril. 58:465-483.

120. Perreault, S.D. (1989) Impaired gamete function: implications for reproductive toxicology. In: Working, P.K. Toxicology of the Male and Female Reproductive Systems. Hemisphere, New York. pp. 217-229.

Chapter 9
Genotoxicity Assessment

Introduction

Genotoxicity describes the destructive effects on the integrity of the genetic material of the cell (DNA or RNA). The agents causing genotoxicity are known as *genotoxins*. So, *genotoxicity* is the ability of genotoxins to cause genetic damage [1]. Before discussing the effects and mechanisms of genotoxicity, it is necessary to clear how the integrity of genetic material is maintained in the cell. The transfer of genetic information within the biological system is a highly regulated process, first stated by Francis Crick in 1957 as "Central dogma of molecular biology". It deals with the *residue-by-residue* sequential transfer of genomic information form DNA to RNA and then to proteins. However, it is not always true as there are some exceptions where DNA can also be synthesized from RNA by the process of reverse transcription like in retroviruses. Generally DNA serves as the genetic material in living organisms except in some cases like RNA viruses where RNA is copied from RNA. DNA can be copied to DNA by the process of 'replication', copied to mRNA by 'transcription' and proteins synthesized by using information stored in mRNA by 'translation'. So, the flow of genetic information in biological system is clearly described by Figure 9.1.

Organisms are prone to the variable degree of endogenous and exogenous DNA insults leading to DNA damage which are precisely managed by DNA-damage checkpoints and DNA repair pathways. The endogenous factors include oxidation, hydrolysis, base mismatch, alkylation *etc.* and exogenous factors includes various environmental factors like radiations and chemicals *etc.* [2]. DNA repair pathways play a crucial role to cope up with DNA damages at the cellular level. The major pathways include the direct reversal pathway, mismatch repair (MMR) pathway, nucleotide excision repair (NER) pathway, base excision repair (BER) pathway, homologous recombination (HR) pathway, and non-homologous end joining (NHEJ) pathway (Figure 9.2). Direct repair system directly acts on the damaged nucleotide

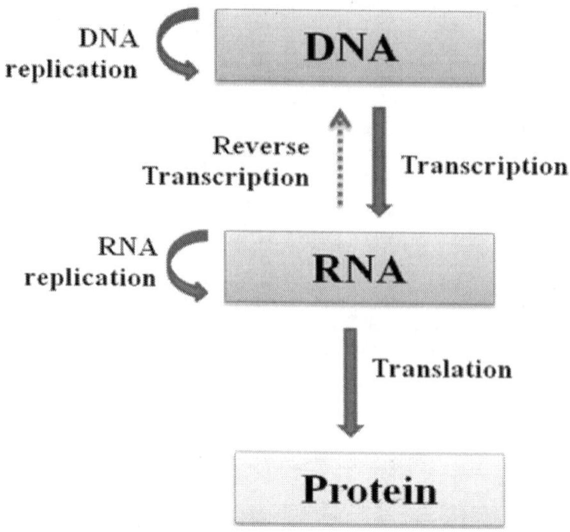

Figure 9.1: Flow of Fenetic Information (Central Dogma).

base and revert it back to the original structure. Only a few nucleotide damages can be repaired through this mechanism. The repair UV mediated pyrimidines dimers is an example of direct repair where repair is facilitated by light dependent direct system called photoreactivation. The base excision repair involves the removal of damaged base and excision of short polynucleotide piece and its resynthesis by DNA polymerase. Nucleotide excision repair is quite similar to base excision repair but it does not involve removal of damaged base. It includes breaking of phophodiester bond on either sides of the same strand creating gap which is repaired by repair system. Xeroderma pigmentosum and Cockayne syndrome in humans are caused due to genetically defective nucleotide excision repair system. The mismatch repair mechanism includes an enzyme system which detect the mismatches occurred during replication, recognize them, excise the incorrect base and repair it through synthesis and ligation. Homologous recombination involves the repair process in which the gap is filled by retrieving a homologous single strand from the other double stranded DNA. On the other hand NHEJ is operated in case of double stranded break where broken ends are directly ligated to non homologous sequence [3].

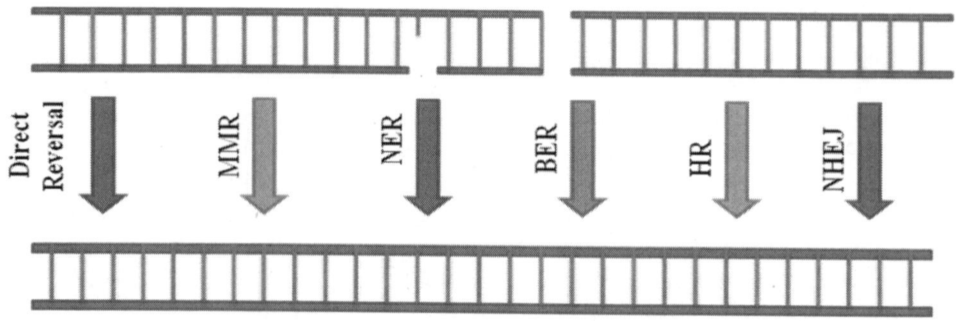

Figure 9.2: Major DNA Repair Pathways.

It has been noticed that genotoxicity is often confused with mutagenicity but there is a considerable difference the two terms. All mutagens are genotoxins but vice versa is not true. The genotoxins which are able to cause mutations in DNA or genome are called mutagens and their ability to cause mutations is known as mutagenicity. The mutations may be spontaneous or induced. Spontaneous mutations are generally caused by errors in the fundamental biological processes like DNA replication or spontaneous errors while induced mutations are caused by the environmental mutagenic agents [4]. So, induction of mutagenicity is one of the effects of genotoxins. Based on the effects, genotoxins are categorized in the following classes:

1. Cancer causing agents or carcinogens
2. Mutation causing agents or mutagens
3. Congenital abnormality causing agents or teratogens

All of the above mentioned effects are mediated through the permanent changes caused in the DNA sequence or its structural or functional integrity.

Mechanism of Genotoxicity

If we look on the molecular mechanism of genotoxicity, the genotoxins act by two ways: Direct and indirect. The first mechanism involves direct attachment of genotoxins to DNA sequencing causing DNA sequence alteration, strand break or chromosomal aberrations. The effects like deletions, breaks and rearrangements are more common at some spots known as *fragile sites* [5]. The indirect mechanism involves the effect of genotoxins on non-DNA targets like enzymes or components of DNA repair pathway, cell cycle regulation or apoptosis. All of these effects cause damage to genome causing genomic instability leading to lethal effects like cell death (Figure 9.3).

Mutation

The agents causing mutations (mutagens) are chemical or physical agents that enhance the occurrence of mutations. The examples of physical mutagens includes the ionizing (*E.g.* X-ray, β-ray) and non ionizing radiations (*e.g.* UV rays). The X ray induced mutation was first described by H.J. Muller in *Drosophila melanogaster*. The direct effects of radiations are caused by directly interaction of radiation energy with DNA while indirect effects are caused due to interaction of DNA with reactive species formed by radiations. The effects of ionizing radiations are very lethal depending on its type and intensity. It may cause the breaking of strands that causes chromosomal breakage which is known as **clastogenic effect** and the agents causing the effect are called **clastogenic agents**. The chemical mutagens includes the base analogs (*e.g.* 5-bromouracil, 2 aminopurine), deaminating agents (*e.g.* nitrous acid), alkylating agents (*e.g.* Nitrogen mustard gas or Ethyl Methane Sulfonate, Methyl Methane Sulfonate, Nitrosoguanidine and dimethylnitrosamine) and intercalating agents (*e.g.* Ethidium bromide, acridine orange and proflavin) [6]. Mutations those incorporated in the somatic cells are termed as **somatic mutations** and the mutations occurring in germ line cells are called **germinal mutations** which pass from one generation to the next.

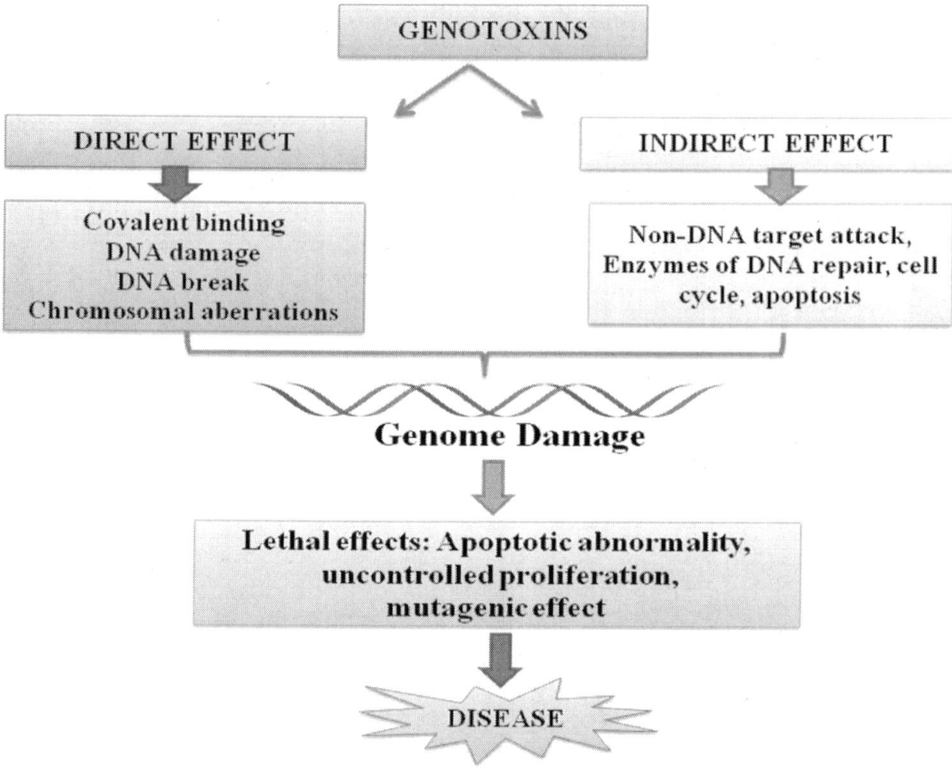

Figure 9.3: Effects of Genotoxins.

Chromosomal aberrations: The integrity of the genome is essential for the survival of multicellular organisms at cellular level. The chromosomal breakdown and its improper segregation during cell cycle are some of the deleterious effects caused by clastogenic genotoxins leading to change in chromosomal number called chromosomal aberrations. This ability of genotoxic substances is also termed as aneugenicity and such genotoxins are known as aneugens. Cancer therapy using genotoxic anticancer agents and radiations is one of the most common exogenous factor causing chromosomal defects. These effects are mediated by two types of mechanisms, DNA reactive mode of action and DNA non-reactive mode [7]. The DNA reactive genotoxins cause damage to DNA leading to double stranded breaks. The excessive DNA damage causes the accumulation of lesions which cannot be corrected by DNA repair system leading to loss of chromosomal elements. The DNA non-reactive mechanism involves the inhibition of DNA synthesis, production of reactive oxygen species and inhibition of spindle formation. The spindle inhibitory effect causes the numerical defect in chromosomes (Aneugenicity) which is most common form of genomic instability (causing aneuploidy) in cancers where anticancer agents (*e.g.* Taxanes and vinca alkaloids) inhibiting assembly or disassembly of spindle tubulin are used for treatment [8].

Apoptosis

Till now we have discussed that DNA is the potential target for most, but not all the genotoxins. DNA damage-triggered programmed cell death or apoptosis is one of the major consequences of genotoxicity and the apoptotic effects have been studied by the use of DNA repair deficient cell lines. However, apoptosis can also be induced by the factors other than those targeting DNA like various physiological stimuli targeting membrane receptors or endogenous mitochondrial damage pathway. The apoptotic responses in the cell lines deficient in the DNA repair pathways like MMR, BER and NER have been studied extensively to rule out the effect of genotoxins on genome. It has been demonstrated by various studies that the DNA repair deficient cells are more prone to apoptosis or hypersensitive to the genotoxins. p53 is the tumor suppressor protein which is a key player in the apoptosis response to the genotoxins. Under normal conditions p53 levels are maintained at low concentration due to short half life of the polypeptide. The DNA damage causes p53 gene to activate leading to rapid increase in its levels and increased ability of p53 to bind DNA to mediate transcriptional activation. This causes activation of a number of genes whose products trigger apoptosis, cell-cycle arrest or DNA repair [9]. It has been found that these regulations are the results of various chemical and enzymatic modifications on p53 like its phosphorylation, de-phosphorylation and acetylation [10].

Cancer

If we see the molecular basis of carcinogenesis, it is augmented by the two means; first is through the gain of oncogenes and other is by the loss of tumor suppressor genes. Proto-oncogenes are the normal genes those help cell to grow normally. These genes code for the proteins responsible for normal cell growth and cell division. If an error (mutation) occur in proto-oncogens, they turned to the defective or malfunctioning gene called oncogenes, whose products causes the conversion of a normal cell to a cancerous cells. Oncogenes are activated by various changes like mutations, gene amplification and chromosomal rearrangements. So, oncogenes are the mutated forms of the proto-oncogenes but not all oncogenes arise from proto-oncogens [11]. Cancer is a multistage event chiefly divided into initiation, promotion, and progression stage occurs over a period of time in the condition of chronic exposure to a carcinogen (Figure 9.4). The normal cell is converted to an initiated cell by the initiation process and the initiating agents are mutagenic with irreversible and additive effect. The initiated cell is converted to preneoplastic or benign lesions by promotion process which can further be converted to a malignant tumor by progression. Some common initiating agents include polycyclic aromatic hydrocarbons present in soot, coal tar and tobacco-specific nitrosamine *etc.* [12]. The examples of promoting agents include the phorbol ester (TPA), benzoyl peroxide, and chrysarobin [13]. Continuous oxidative stress and chronic inflammation mediated by cytokines, chemokines, and eicosanoids promote tumor progression. Some irritating agents like UV light and tobacco smoke also exhibit tumor promoting activity [14].

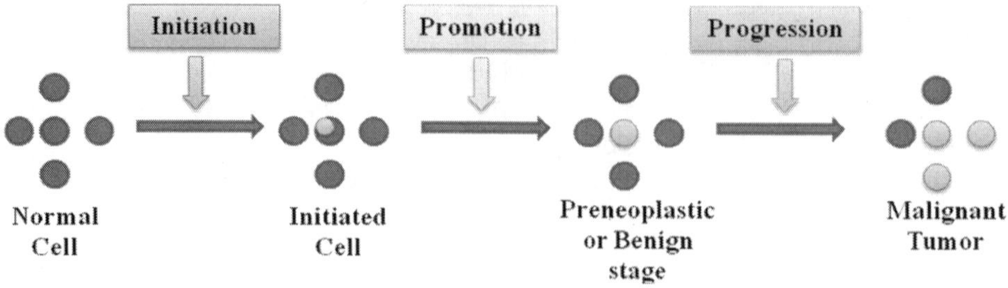

Figure 9.4: Stages of Cancer Progression.

Ras, *HER2* and *myc* genes are well known oncogenes. *Ras* encoding intracellular signal-transduction protein was the first proto-oncogene to be reported to turn out to be an oncogene through point mutation in the case of several pancreatic, lung, colon and thyroid tumors [15]. Many females with breast cancer have gene amplification mutation in *HER2* gene which encodes the protein receptors involved in growth and division of breast cells [16]. *Myc* gene is associated with a cancerous condition called Burkitt's lymphoma and transformed to oncogene through chromosomal translocation [17].

Apart from oncogenes, tumor suppressor genes are another key players in cancer regulation by slowing down cell division, repairing DNA mistakes and promoting programmed cell death. The important difference in oncogene and tumor suppressor genes is that oncogenes cause cancer when they are *activated* or *turned on* from proto-oncogenes, but tumor suppressor genes cause cancer when they are *inactivated* or *turned off*. In more than half of the human cancers defect in p53 gene encoding p53 protein has been found. *BRCA1* and *BRCA2* are important tumor suppressor genes, whom mutation increases the risk of hereditary breast and ovarian cancer in women [18].

Teratogenic Effects

The agents causing birth defects or congenital anomalies are termed as teratogens. Several teratogenic agents like ionizing radiation and xenobiotics (*E.g.* phenytoin, benzo[a]pyrene, thalidomide) can initiate the formation of reactive oxygen species (ROS) that causes oxidative damage to DNA causing genotoxicity [19]. Oxidative damage is more likely to occur through altered gene transcription rather than through incorporation of genetic mutations. Ionizing radiation can cause the injury to developing embryo by causing cell death or chromosomal damage. 8–15 week period after fertilization is the most critical exposure period to radiation and the developing central nervous system (CNS) is most sensitive to the damage [20].

Genotoxicity Testing

Genotoxicity testing involves the methods or assays developed to assess the chemicals' potential to cause DNA damage. These tests have a considerable role in the identification of hazardous effects of therapeutic drugs, toxins, nanomaterials, cosmetics, agrochemicals, environmental pollutants, industrial wastes and food additives for regulatory purposes. Various *in vitro* and *in vivo* genotoxicity assays have been developed over a period of time which can be implemented in bacterial, yeast and mammalian cells. The *in vitro* assays are more suitable for detection of primary genotoxicity where as the in *vivo tests* are suitable to assess the secondary genotoxic effects via inflammation and oxidative stress. The biggest challenge in testing genotoxicity is the reliability and sensitivity of the particular assay to detect the various DNA damage lesions and cellular responses to genotoxins. The main limitation in the genotoxicity evaluation methods is the false positive results which challenge the reliability of an assay. There is no single assay at present which can solve all the issues and give satisfactory results [21,22]. Therefore a set or battery of assays is generally applied for effective genotoxicity testing. There are several regulatory guidelines or standards established for genotoxicity testing. The advancement in molecular biology tools, cell culture, genomics, and gene expression analysis made it more effective to test the genotoxicity. The current genotoxicity assays includes Ames test, micronucleus (MN) test, comet assay, sister chromatid exchange (SCE) test, Mouse Lymphoma Test, SOS chromo test and chromosomal aberration test [21, 22].

Ames Test

This test is also known as bacterial reverse mutation assay and is most widely used assay developed by Bruce Ames is 1970s. It uses the different auxotrophic mutants of *Salmonella typhimurium* and *E.coli* carrying defective gene for essential amino acid synthesis. The induction of reverse mutation in the bacterial strains causes reversal of mutagenic effect is the basis of this test (Figure 9.5). The classical Ames test uses several strains of *salmonella typhimurium* and *E.coli* carrying mutations in genes required for histidine or tryptophan amino acid biosynthesis. So the strains require histidine for growth because they cannot produce it. In case of *Salmonella* TA97, TA98, TA100, TA102, TA104, TA1535, TA1537, and TA1538 strains used as the tester stains and Escherichia coli WP2 and WP2urvA tester strains carrying a defective or mutant gene are used [23]. The mutagenic agent causes the reverse

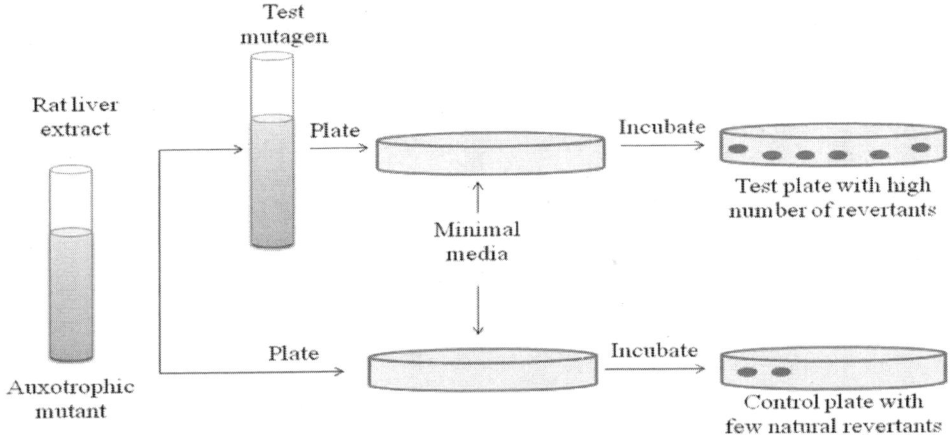

Figure 9.5: Ames Test.

mutation in the mutant strains which cause their resumption to wild type produce essential amino acids. The bacteria now grow as the visible colonies on minimal medium. The number of colonies is taken as the direct measure of mutagenicity of the test compound. Although the test is most widely used test in the genotoxic studies but there are some disadvantages of this method. It is difficult to detect the genotoxins which do not cause frame-shift or point mutation. It has also been noticed that sometime the toxins are not cause genotoxicity directly but their metabolites are responsible to genotoxic effects. Since *Salmonella* and *E. coli* are prokaryotes, so the Ames test is not a perfect model for genotoxicity testing in animals or humans. However the similar test has been designed using human liver S9 fraction [24].

Micronucleus Test (MNT)

Micronucleus test is the important test used for the screening of genotoxins by evaluating the presence of micronuclei. Micronuclei, also known as Howell Jolly bodies were first identified by William Howell and Justin Jolly in the cytoplasm of erythrocytes as the fragments of nuclear materials. These micronuclei are formed during the anaphase stage of mitosis or meiosis. The fragments of chromosomes do not move to the opposite poles due to improper attachment to the spindle fibre leading to their miss incorporation in the daughter nuclei. These dislocated chromosomal fragments acquire a nuclear membrane which gives them the appearance like a small nucleus at staining called as micronuclei (Figure 9.6). The scoring of micronuclei is a reliable assay for the assessment of genotoxicity induced through the excessive DNA breakage at chromosomal level leading to genomic instability, chromosomal aberration and aneuploidy [25].

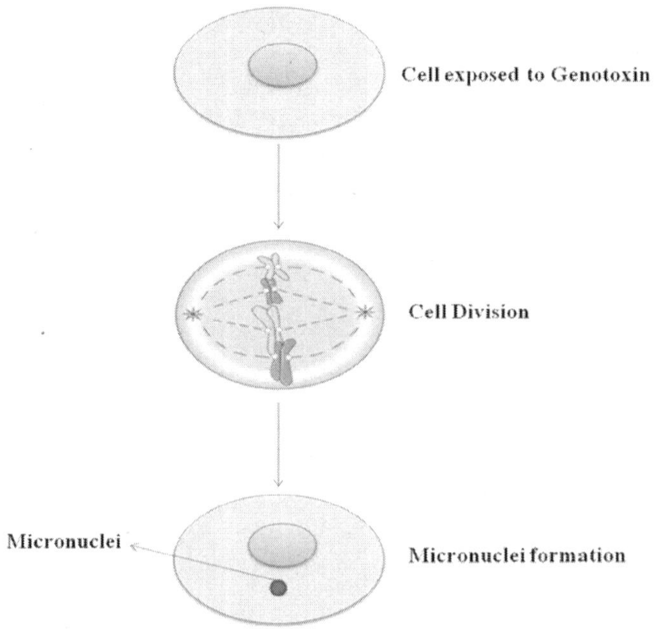

Figure 9.6: Micronucleus Test.

Comet Assay

The comet assay or single-cell gel electrophoresis (SCGE) described by Ostling and Johanson is the simple method to measure DNA strand breaks in eukaryotic cell. This assay is a widely used test for determination of nucleotide base damage, single or double DNA strand break in almost all the species. The test can easily be applied on any eukaryotic cell population *in vitro, in vivo,* or *ex vivo.* The procedure of comet assay involves three steps: Encapsulation, lysis and electrophoresis. The cells derived from *in vivo* and *in vitro* genotoxin exposed cultures are subjected to encapsulation into Agarose layered on a microscopic slide. The embedded cells are then lysed by using high salt and detergent, which causes elimination of membrane, soluble cellular components and histones. The DNA remains in the form of nucleoid containing supercoiled loops linked to nuclear matrix. The breakage in DNA causes relaxation of supercoiling leading to formation of "comet tail" like extended patterns under fluorescent microscopy after electrophoresis. The breakage efficiency can be easily correlated to the intensity of comet tail [26]. Certain software tools are also available for the scoring of comet tail through automatized image analysis.

Chromosomal Aberration Test (CAT)

Chromosomal aberration is one of the important biomarker of genotoxicity mediated by structural chromosome change, chromatid breakage and translocation. CAT can be used to study the effect of genotoxic agents both *in vitro* and *in vivo* formats by using cultured cells and whole organisms respectively. The genotoxin treated cells are incubated with metaphase inhibitor like colchicine. The aberration finally determined by visualizing the chromosomes under microscope using suitable staining procedure. The number of cells carrying aberrations can be taken as the degree of clastogenicity [27].

SCE Test

The SCE test stands for sister chromatid exchange test. The method relies upon the cytogenetic monitoring of human peripheral lymphocytes exposed to chemical mutagens. SCE occurs in S phase of cell cycle where double strand break takes place followed by exchange of whole DNA duplex. It is induced by genotoxic agents causing double stranded DNA breaks and errors in DNA replication. In SCE test, the mammalian cells are treated with genotoxic agent and allowed to grow for two replication cycles in presence of media containing 5-Bromo-2-deoxyuridine (5-BrdU). After that the cells are treated with spindle inhibitor like colchicine to arrest the cell in metaphase and visualized using fluorescence plus Giemsa (FPG) procedure [28].

Miscellaneous Methods and Future Possibilities

Apart from the above listed tests there are some other tests reported to be used for the determination of genotoxicity. Unscheduled DNA synthesis (UDS) test, SOS chromotest and somatic mutation and recombination test (SMART) are the other less known test used in the genotoxicity studies. The advancement in molecular biology is making the genotoxicity testing more easy, rapid and reliable. Transgenic rodent (TGR) mutation models are now available for the in-vivo genotoxicity assessment

[29]. The latest techniques including next generation high throughput sequencing and analysis tools and global gene expression analysis using microarray or DNA chips can be effectively used in genotoxicity analysis and related studies [30,31].

REFERENCES

1. Nagarathna, P. K. M., M. Johnson Wesley, P. Sriram Reddy, Reena. K. 2013. Review on Genotoxicity, its Molecular Mechanisms and Prevention. *Int. J. Pharm. Sci. Rev. Res.*, 22(1): 43, 236-243
2. Srivastava, R., Mishra, N., Singh, U. M. and Srivastava, R. 2016. Genotoxicity: mechanisms and its impact on human diseases. *Octa J. Biosci.* 4(2): 67-70.
3. Clancy, S. 2008. DNA damage and repair: mechanisms for maintaining DNA integrity. *Nature Education.* 1(1): 103
4. Griffiths AJF, Miller JH, Suzuki DT, *et al.*, 2000. An Introduction to Genetic Analysis. 7th edition. New York: W. H. Freeman.
5. Ma, K., Qiu, L., Mrasek, K., *et al.*, 2012. Common fragile sites: genomic hotspots of DNA damage and carcinogenesis. *Int J Mol Sci.* 13(9): 11974–11999. doi: 10.3390/ijms130911974
6. Miller, E. C. and Miller, J. A. 1971. The Mutagenicity of Chemical Carcinogens: Correlations, Problems, and Interpretations. In: Hollaender A. (eds) Chemical Mutagens. Springer, Boston, MA. Pp 83-119.
7. Jain, A. K., Singh, D., Dubey, K., Maurya, R. and Pandey, A. K. 2018. Chromosomal Aberrations. In Mutagenicity: Assays and Applications. Academic Press. Pp. 69-92, ISBN 9780128092521. https: //doi.org/10.1016/B978-0-12-809252-1.00004-3.
8. Vargas-Rondón, N., Villegas, V. E. and Rondón-Lagos, M. 2017. The Role of Chromosomal Instability in Cancer and Therapeutic Responses. *Cancers. 10*(1): 4. https: //doi.org/10.3390/cancers10010004.
9. Haupt, S., Berger, M., Goldberg, Z. and Haupt, Y. 2003. Apoptosis- the p53 network. Journal of Cell Science. 116: 4077-4085. doi: 10.1242/jcs.00739.
10. Kruse, J. P. and Gu, W. 2009. Modes of p53 regulation. *Cell.* 137(4): 609–622. doi: 10.1016/j.cell.2009.04.050.
11. Koeffler, H. P., McCormick, F. and Denny, C. 1991. Molecular mechanisms of cancer. *West J Med.* 1991; 155(5): 505–514.
12. Basu, A. K. 2018. DNA Damage, Mutagenesis and Cancer. *Int J Mol Sci.* 19(4): 970. doi: 10.3390/ijms19040970
13. John DiGiovanni. 1992. Multistage carcinogenesis in mouse skin. Pharmacology and Therapeutics. 54 (1): 63-128. https: //doi.org/10.1016/0163-7258(92)90051-Z.
14. Soehnge, H., Ouhtit, A. and Ananthaswamy, O. N. 1997. Mechanisms of induction of skin cancer by UV radiation. *Front Biosci.* 2: d538-51.
15. Pappou, E. P., and Ahuja, N. 2010. The role of oncogenes in gastrointestinal cancer. Gastrointestinal cancer research : GCR, (Suppl 1), S2–S15.

16. Iqbal, N. and Iqbal, N. 2014. Human Epidermal Growth Factor Receptor 2 (HER2) in Cancers: Overexpression and Therapeutic Implications. *Molecular Biology International*. 852748. doi. http: //dx.doi.org/10.1155/2014/852748.

17. Nguyen, L., Papenhausen, P., and Shao, H. 2017. The Role of c-MYC in B-Cell Lymphomas: Diagnostic and Molecular Aspects. *Genes*. 8(4): 116. doi. https: //doi.org/10.3390/genes8040116

18. Mehrgou, A., and Akouchekian, M. 2016. The importance of BRCA1 and BRCA2 genes mutations in breast cancer development. *Medical journal of the Islamic Republic of Iran*. 30: 369.

19. Wells, P. G., McCallum, G. P., Chen, C. S., Henderson, J. T., Lee, C. J. J., Perstin, J., Preston, T. J., Wiley, M. J. and Wong, A. W. 2009. Oxidative Stress in Developmental Origins of Disease: Teratogenesis, Neurodevelopmental Deficits, and Cancer. *Toxicological Sciences*. 108(1): 4–18, https: //doi.org/10.1093/toxsci/kfn263

20. Enid Gilbert-Barness. 2010. Teratogenic Causes of Malformations. *Annals of Clinical and Laboratory Science*.40(2): 99-114.

21. Turkez, H., Arslan, M. E. and Ozdemir, O. 2017.Genotoxicity testing: progress and prospects for the next decade. *Expert Opinion on Drug Metabolism and Toxicology*. DOI: 10.1080/17425255.2017.1375097

22. Mohamed, S., Sabita, U., Rajendra, S., Raman, D. 2017. Genotoxicity: Mechanisms, Testing Guidelines and Methods. *Glob. J. Pharmaceu. Sci.* 1(5): 555575. DOI: 10.19080/GJPPS.2017.02.555575

23. Ames, B. N, Lee, F. D. and Durston, W. E. 1973. An improved bacterial test system for the detection and classification of mutagens and carcinogens. *Proceedings of the National Academy of Sciences of the United States of America*. **70** (3): 782–786.

24. Hakura, A., Shimada, H., Nakajima, M., Sui, H., Kitamoto, S., Suzuki, S. and Satoh, T. 2005. Salmonella/human S9 mutagenicity test: a collaborative study with 58 compounds. Mutagenesis. 20(3): 217-28.

25. Hayashi M. 2016. The micronucleus test-most widely used in vivo genotoxicity test. *Genes Environ*. 38: 18. doi: 10.1186/s41021-016-0044-x.

26. Azqueta, A. and Dusinska, M. 2015. The use of the comet assay for the evaluation of the genotoxicity of nanomaterials. *Frontiers in genetics*. 6: 239. doi. https: //doi.org/10.3389/fgene. 2015.00239.

27. Kirkland, D. 1998. Chromosome aberration testing in genetic toxicology—past, present and future. In Mutation Research/Fundamental and Molecular Mechanisms of Mutagenesis. 404(1–2): 173-185. ISSN 0027-5107. https: //doi.org/10.1016/S0027-5107(98)00111-0.

28. Jain, A. K., Singh, D., Dubey, K., Maurya, R., Mittal, S. and Pandey, A. K. 2018. Models and Methods for *In vitro* Toxicity. In *In vitro* Toxicology. Academic Press. pp. 45-65. ISBN 9780128046678. doi 10.1016/B978-0-12-804667-8.00003-1.

29. Boverhof, D. R., Chamberlain, M. P., Elcombe, C. R., Gonzalez, F. J., Heflich, R. H., Hernández, L. G., Jacobs, A. C., Jacobson-Kram, D., Luijten, M., Maggi, A., Manjanatha, M. G., Benthem, J. V. and Gollapudi, B. B. 2011. Transgenic Animal Models in Toxicology: Historical Perspectives and Future Outlook, *Toxicological Sciences*. 121(2): 207–233. doi. https: //doi.org/10.1093/toxsci/kfr075

30. Newton, R. K., Aardema, M. and Aubrecht, J. 2004. The utility of DNA microarrays for characterizing genotoxicity. *Environ Health Perspect*. 112(4): 420–422. doi: 10.1289/ehp.6709

31. Powell, J., Bennett, M., Evans, K. *et al.*, 2015. 3D-DIP-Chip: A microarray-based method to measure genomic DNA damage. *Sci Rep* 5: 7975. doi https: //doi.org/10.1038/srep07975.

Chapter 10

Immunoassays

Immunoassays are a bioanalytical method to study the quantification of an analyte based on the reaction between the analyte and a specific protein against the analyte. The basic principle behind the working of these assays is the binding reaction between a certain amount of labeled analyte and a variable amount of unlabelled sample analyte on to the binding sites of a highly specific anti-analyte antibody. The reaction complex formed is incubated to facilitate the binding of analytes to the antibody, followed by removal of the unbound using physical or chemical methods. The activity (radiation, fluorescence, or enzyme-substrate reaction) of the complex is quantitatively measured in either bound or unbound fraction and based on activity; a standard curve is plotted with the signal generated against variable concentrations of the analytes. This calibrated curve obtained can further be used to measure the activity of an unknown analyte. These labeled analytes are designed in such a way to detect very small quantities (up to femtomole and attomole) of the analyte that too with high sensitivity in complex systems. The first immunoassay was developed using radiolabelled insulin by Yalow and Berson in the year 1959. The radiolabelled insulin was used by them for the assessment of insulin concentration in human plasma.

The establishment of a drug immunoassay includes the competitive interaction between the drug antigen in the sample and the amount the antigen added as a part of the test system to bind with the antibody. A calibration curve is developed of the set of standards with the known volume of the drug added. The results produced by labeling the antigen or the antibody with a particularly suitable marker helps to generate a signal which is then compared with the above calibration curve.

Antigen-Antibody Interaction

The antibody's affinity to the antigen is defined as the strength of the interaction between the two. The variable arm of the antibody interacts through the non-covalent forces to the sites on the antigen. The various forces involved are hydrophobic bonds, hydrogen bonds, Van der Waals forces, and electrostatic forces. Avidity (combined strength of multiple affinities) marks a better measure to study the antigen-antibody interaction. Three factors mainly responsible for avidity are:

1. The affinity of the antibody epitope
2. Valency of the antigen and the antibody
3. The structural arrangement of the interacting portions

Antigen-antibody interaction is a bimolecular reversible interaction. Various factors affects the antigen-antibody interaction, such as temperature, pH, ionic strength, the concentration of antigen and antibody, number of antigen sites per cell, duration of incubation of the antigen and the antibody.

Labels Used in Immunoassays

Various types of agents used as labels are employed in immunological assays. These may include:

1. **Radioactive compounds**: Different radioactive compounds are used for the labeling of the antigen. These may include: ^{125}I, ^{3}H, ^{75}Se *etc.* The radioactivity emitted by the antigen-antibody interaction can be easily detected, and this forms the basis of radioimmunoassay. But in this, there are some problems associated like: health hazards produced by the emitted radioactivity, high cost of the instrument facility, the short half-life of the radioactive isotope and the requirement a trained handler.
2. **Enzymes**: These mark the most widely and commonly used label for antigens in immunoassays. The use of these enzymes helps in the development of color after the antigen-antibody interaction in the presence of a certain specific substrate. The optical density after the final reaction is measured and results can be obtained. Various enzymes used for this include Horse Radish peroxidase, Alkaline phosphatase, Glucose oxidase, β-D-Galactosidase, β-D-Glucose oxidase, *etc.*[1].
3. **Fluorescent compounds**: These compounds (*e.g.* Luciferase peroxidase) absorb light or energy of a specific wavelength and then emits the wave of a certain wavelength which is detected by the detection system.
4. **Chemiluminescent substance**: These substances help to convert a substrate to a reaction product which then emit a photon of light (luminescent material), which is then detected by a luminescent signal instrument *i.e.*, it is the light produced out of a chemical reaction. It can be of three types: labeled chemical directly emitting a light photon, enzyme-catalyzed emission of a light photon and redox reaction mediated emission of a light photon.

Use of Immunoassays for Pharmaceutical Analysis

Immunoassays find a wide range of applications in various pharmaceutical procedures such as:

- ☆ Drug monitoring,
- ☆ Disease diagnosis,
- ☆ Clinical-pharmacokinetic analysis
- ☆ Bioequivalence studies in case of discovery of drugs
- ☆ In the pharmaceutical industry

They are used in various pharmaceutical analysis due to its property of analysis of biological analytes with high specificity and sensitivity. They are also extremely beneficial in the analysis of high-throughput data.

General Approach to Carry Out Immunological Assays in Pharmacology

There are four requirements to carry out the immunoassays. These are the antibody (may be polyclonal or monoclonal), labels (radioisotope, enzyme, *etc.*), the separation matrices (secondary antibody, microbeads, charcoal, polyethylene glycol) and an instrumentation facility (spectrophotometer, fluorimeter, gamma counter).

There are various steps in the development of a drug immunoassay[2]:

1. Taking into account all the indications for the development of an appropriate immunoassay.
2. Preparation and organization of all the reagents required to carry out the assay.
    - ☆ Selection of a label
    - ☆ Selection of the animals and their immunization schedule for antibody production
    - ☆ Requirement of immunogens
    - ☆ Selection of phase separation (if required)
3. Verifying and affirming the developed immunoassay technically
    - ☆ Proper understanding of antigen-antibody interaction dynamics and optimization
    - ☆ Analysis of the assays' sensitivity and specificity
    - ☆ Assessment of the accuracy and repeatability of the assay
    - ☆ Quality control of the assay
4. Implementation and utilization of the immunoassay:
    - ☆ Understanding the limitations of the assay
    - ☆ A detailed analysis of pharmacodynamics and pharmacokinetics of the drug in the trial in subjects and patients
    - ☆ Proper recognition of toxicological problems
    - ☆ The exact judgment of the therapeutic dose range to be administered

Categories of Immunoassays

Immunoassays can be classified in various ways. The first classification is based on the use of labeled proteins. Few assays use unlabelled agents like immunodiffusion and nephelometry and the other uses labeled groups (radioisotopes, enzymes *etc.*) like radio-immunoassay and enzyme immunoassay. Based on separation of the antigen-antibody complexes, those assays that require the uncoupling of the antigen-antibody complex are mentioned as heterogeneous (separative) immunoassay and those that do not require the uncoupling are referred as a homogenous (non-separative) assay. These heterogeneous and homogenous assays may also be divided into competitive and non-competitive assays. In competitive immunoassays, the unlabeled analyte competes with a labeled analyte in the assay. It can be antigen-capture immunoassay or antibody capture immunoassay. Whereas, in non-competitive immunoassay the unlabelled analyte is allowed to bind in the presence of an excess of the labeled analyte. Talking about labeled immunoassays, they may be categorized into five types, namely- Radioimmunoassay (RIA), Counting Immunoassay (CIA), Enzyme-Linked Immunosorbent Assay (ELISA), Fluoroimmunoassay (FIA) and Chemiluminescenceimmunoassay (CLI). It is worth mentioning that there is currently a movement towards developing label-free immunoassays. Basically in general, almost all immunoassays are established under the concept of the interaction of a target molecule (antigen) with a complementary antibody.

Types of Immunoassays

The development of immunoassays has revolutionized the field of disease diagnosis, therapeutic drug monitoring, drug discovery studies, and pharmaceutical industries. Initially pharmacology was mainly concerned with pharmacodynamics (what drugs do to the body) but advances in these bioassays led to the extensive study and research on pharmacokinetics (what the body does to the drugs). Drug immunoassays have been efficiently utilized for many research applications[3].

While talking about, these assays, there comes the point whether these assays are specific and efficient in quantifying a test sample. This led to the discovery of the use of labeled immunoassays where the antibody used may be labeled either radio-isotope, fluorescent, enzyme, or chemiluminescent agent. These labeled assays are so much versatile so that they can handle a few to thousand samples per day that too in a single go. The history of using the labeled assay system started long ago in 1959 when for the first time, Yalow and Berson used radiolabeled insulin to evaluate the concentration of insulin in human plasma and thus, the first radioimmunoassay (RIA) was developed. Following this, in 1971, Engvail and Perlman used an enzyme-linked anti-immunoglobin antibody to detect the concentration of antibody which led to the discovery of the first ELISA.

RIA

RIA was the primogenitor of the various heterogeneous immunoassays. The system of RIA consists of a sample containing an antigen of interest, a complementary

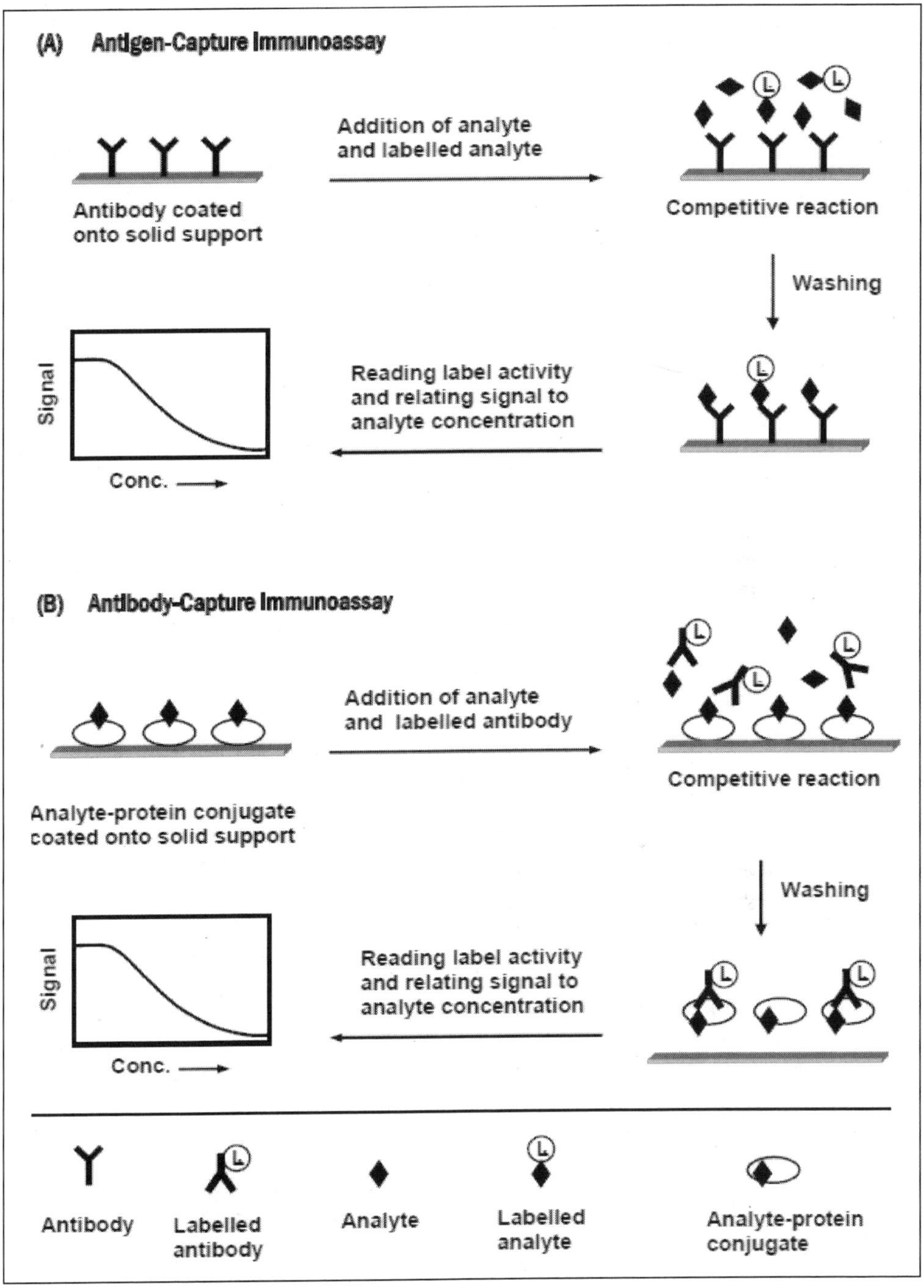

Figure 10.1: Competitive Immunoassay.

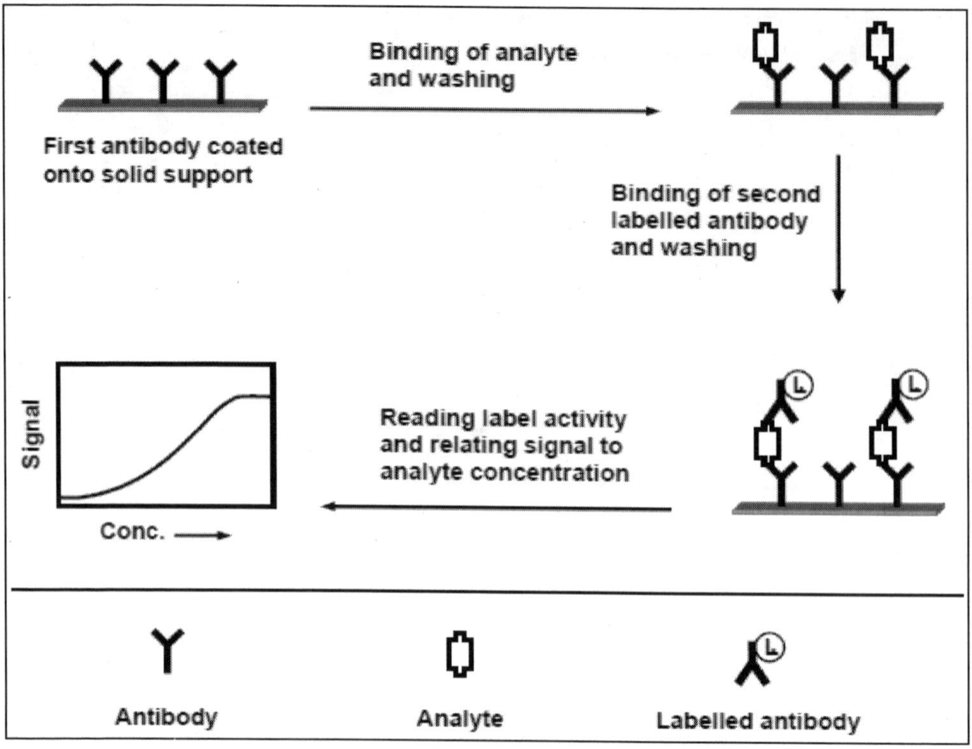

Figure 10.2: Non-competitive Immunoassay.

antibody and a radiolabeled antigen. First, the sample antigen and antibody are subjected to incubation so that both antigen and antibody can interact. Following this, the radiolabeled antigen is added that competes with the sample antigen and displaces it from the antibody. The amount of samples antigen is inversely related to the amount of radiolabeled antigen. A second antibody directed against the primary antibody is mixed to the system that flocculates the solution which further facilitates the separation of the primary antibody from the solution. On centrifuging this solution, an antigen-antibody pellet is obtained that is checked for the amount of radiolabeled antigen present in the system. The most important advantage of RIA is that it can measure compounds in biological fluids with high precision and extreme sensitivity. Difficulties associated with the handling and storage of radioactivity, disposal of radioactive waste and the half-life of the radioactive labels have resulted in RIA being replaced largely by non-isotopic immunoassay methods.

RIA is the oldest type of immunoassay wherein a radioisotope is coupled to an antigen of interest and then bound with its complementary antibody. Then the sample antigen is added that competes with the radioactive antigens to attach to the antibody. After washing away the unbound antigens the radioactivity of samples is measured which is inversely related to the amount of target antigen. But the health hazards due to the usage of radioactive substances led to the thought of using something harmless and favourable to the environment.

Counting Immunoassay

Polystyrene beads are coated with many antibodies complementary to the target antigen and incubated to allow the beads to bind to multiple antigens and group together into a large mass. Then the entire solution is passed through a cell counter which measures only unbound beads and their count is inversely related to the amount of antigen.

Enzyme-Linked Immunosorbent Assay

In this assay the antibody is linked to an enzyme and after incubation, with antigen the unbound antibody is washed away. The activity of the enzyme-bound antibody is quantified by adding a substrate to the reaction wherein the enzyme catalyzes the reaction to produce a color that is quantified[5].

There are four basic variants of ELISA:

a) **Direct ELISA**: This is the most simple type in which the antigen of interest is added to the ELISA plate and incubated. After its adsorption on the plate surface, it is washed and a blocking agent is added which blocks the remaining binding sites on the plate. Then the antibody bound to an enzyme that is complementary to the antigen is added to the plate and incubated. After incubation, it is again washed properly and the substrate (like θ-phenyl diamine (OPD) or tetramethylbenzidine (TMB) when Horse Radish peroxidase (HRPO) is used as an enzyme) is added which reacts with the present enzyme and produces a colored product and its optical density is measured at a certain specific wavelength.

b) **Indirect ELISA**: This is the type of ELISA that makes use of the anti-antibody, which is bound to the enzyme, unlike the antibody being linked to an enzyme in the case of direct ELISA. In this, the sample antigen is coated onto the wells of the ELISA plate, followed by washing and then blocking the unquenched sites. Again washing the plate, and then the primary antibody is added to the wells and incubated for a certain period to react with the antigen. This is then again followed by washing to remove the unattached antibody. After this, the anti-antibody (conjugate) linked with an enzyme, which will target the F_c region of the antibody, is added to the wells to react with the antibody. After incubation, this is again washed to remove the unattached anti-antibody. Then a suitable substrate is added to the wells, which will react with the enzyme, and a colored product is formed whose O. D. is recorded.

c) **Competitive ELISA**: This is the type of ELISA in which two antigens one the sample antigen and the other similar to this antigen are involved which can bind to the antibody. They both will compete with each other to bind to the same site on the antibody. Mostly biotin is added to the sample antigen so that when the streptavidin protein is added, it binds to biotin, and a signal is generated.

d) **Sandwich ELISA**: This is a type of ELISA in which the antigen is sandwiched between the two complementary antibodies. An antibody

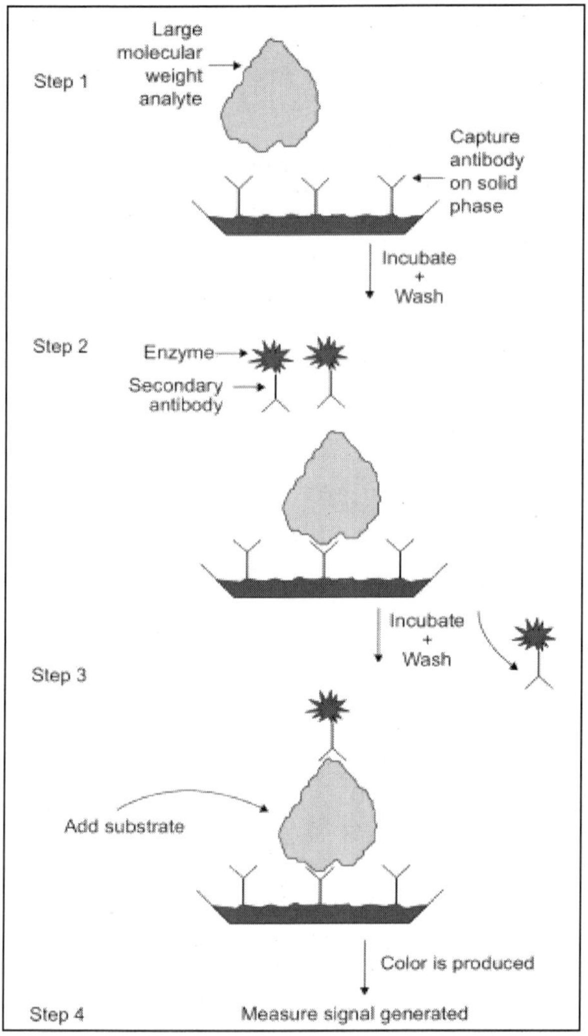

Figure 10.3: The Basic Technique of ELISA (Indirect ELISA).

(capture antibody) is coated to the wells of the ELISA plate. Further after coating, a blocking agent is added to block the unquenched sites. Then the sample antigen is added and incubated to react with the antibody and the washed. The unreacted antigen will be washed out. Then the conjugated antibody is added to the wells and incubated. After incubation, the substrate is added to the wells which react with the enzyme linked to the conjugated antibody and color is developed whose O.D. is measured.

Fluoroimmunoassay

In this assay, the antibody against the analyte is fluorescent-labeled which on incubation interacts with the antigen and the fluorescent intensity is measured. The binding of the antibody leads to some changes in the fluorescence activity of the labeled analyte. The most common type in this type of assay is fluorescent polarization fluoroimmunoassay (FPFIA). This is applied in the field of drug discovery and therapeutic monitoring of various analytes[6]. The excitation of the fluorescent analyte by the polarized light is dependent on the rotational motion of the conjugate and inversely on the decay constant of the probe. Another, Time-resolved fluoroimmunoassay (TRFIA) is used for the analysis of various biological hormones and pharmaceutical compounds. In this, the labels used are chelates of palladium and lanthanide compounds[7].

Chemiluminescence Immunoassay

The basic principle is the same as that of ELISA and Fluoroimmunoassay but here the reported is different. A chemical reaction within the system allows the electron to move to a higher energy state which on returning to its ground state emits the light that is quantified. A magneto-actuated Chemiluminescence assay has been developed to detect the presence of the Zika virus in humans. In pharmacology, it is used for the analysis of compounds such as antiepileptics (Carbamazepine, Phenobarbital, Phenytoin, Valproic acid), bronchodilators (Salbutamol, clenbuterol), vitamins (Vitamin B12), hormones (Insulin, Thyroxine, Estradiol, Testosterone), tumor markers (Prostate-specific antigen)[4].

Lateral Flow Assay (LFA)

This assay is used for the detection of the target analyte in a liquid sample. It has various advantages such as: inexpensive, simple, high specificity, good sensitivity, portable technology, rapid (usually gives result in 5-30 min.). Lateral flow immunoassay can be used to detect either the antibodies or other target analytes such as proteins, hormones, *etc.*[8]. It makes use of a simple adsorbent pad strip on which the liquid sample is applied at an end of the adsorbent strip, the test analyte moves in the strip through capillary action and interacts with the detection system (complementary to the test analyte), which is a colored or fluorescent particle-commonly used are colloidal gold or latex microspheres impregnated in the strip[9].

Advtanges of Immunoassays

1. Highly sensitive technique
2. Highly specific
3. It can be carried out with a minimum amount of the sample
4. Rapid technique
5. A large number of repetitive assays can be performed in a short time

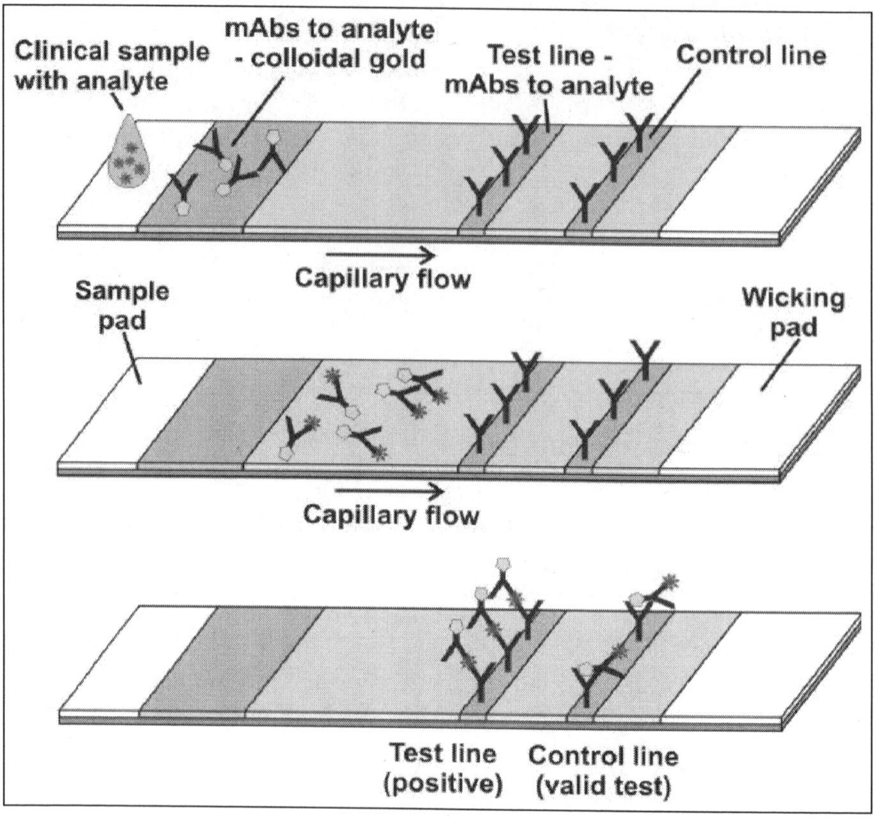

Figure 10.4: Lateral Flow Assay using Colloidal Gold as a Label[10].

Diadvtanges of Immunoassays

1. High initial cost
2. Sometimes technical complexity of the assay
3. Health hazards in case of RIA due to radioactivity

Application of Immunoassays in Pharmacology

The application of immunoassays in pharmacology can be divided into three heads:

1. Therapeutic drug monitoring
2. Experimental pharmacokinetics and clinical pharmacology
3. Forensic, epidemiological, and toxicological analysis

Drug immunoassays find applications in various clinical research like for example, the study of the pharmacokinetics of morphine after it is introduced intravenously and therapeutic drug monitoring of an anti-cancer drug, tegafur, by indirect competitive ELISA[11].

REFERENCES

1. Hempen C. and Karst U. 2006. Labeling strategies for bioassays. Anal Bioanal Chem. **384**: 572–583.
2. Marks V. 1981. Immunoassays in Pharmacology and Toxicology. Immunoassays for the 80s. MTP Press Limited.
3. Moore A. , Bullingham R., McQuay H., Allen M., Baldwin D., Cole A. 1984. Spinal fluid kinetics of morphine and heroin. *Clinical Pharmacology and Therapeutics*. **35**. 40–45.
4. Darwish I.A. 2006. Immunoassay Methods and their Applications in Pharmaceutical Analysis: Basic Methodology and Recent Advances. International Journal *of* Biomedical science. 217-235
5. Grange R.D., Thompson J.P., Lambert D.G. 2014. Radioimmunoassay, enzyme and non-enzyme-based Immunoassays. British Journal of Anesthesia. **112 (2)**: 213–16.
7. Ankelo M., Westerlund A., Ilonen J., Knip M., *et al.*, 2003. *Clin. Chem.* **49**: 908-915.
6. Gomez-Henz A. and Aguilar-Caballos M.P. 2003. *Comb. Chem. High Throughput Screen*. **6**: 177-182.
8. Tian W., Wang L., Lei H., Sun Y., Xiao Z. 2018. Antibody production and application for immunoassay development of environmental hormones: a review. *Chem. Biol. Technol. Agric.* **5**: 5.
9. Koczula K.M. and Gallotta A. 2016. Lateral flow assays. Essays Biochem. **60(1)**: 111–120.
10. Lee L., Nordman E.S., Johnson M.D., Oldham M.F. 2013. A Low-Cost, High-Performance System for Fluorescence Lateral Flow Assays. Biosensors. **3**. 360-373.
11. Broto M., McCabe R., Galve R., Pilar Marco M. 2017. A high throughput immunoassay for the therapeutic drug monitoring of tegafur. Analyst. Issue **13**.

Chapter 11

Computer-Aided Drug Design

Computer-Aided Drug Design (CADD) refers to the application of informatics methods within rational drug design, to discover, design and optimize biologically active compounds. Besides it is a process of drug design with the help of computers that may be used at any of the following stages of drug discovery:

1. HIT identification using virtual screening
2. HIT to Lead optimization of affinity and selectivity
3. Lead optimization: Optimization of other pharmaceutical activities while maintaining affinity.

The pipeline of drug discovery from idea to market consists of seven basic steps [1]

1. Disease selection
2. Target selection
3. Lead compound identification
4. Lead optimization
5. Pre-clinical trial testing
6. Clinical trial testing
7. Pharmacogenomics optimization

The compounds for testing can be obtained from natural sources (plants, animals, microorganisms) and by chemical synthesis. These compounds can be rejected as perspective less owing to absence or low activity, existence of toxicity or carcinogenity, complexity of synthesis, insufficient efficiency, *etc.* [2, 3]. The reduction of time-consuming and cost of the last stages of drug testing is unlikely due to strict state standards on their realization. Therefore main efforts to increasing the efficiency of development of drugs are directed to stages of discovery and optimization of ligands [4]. However, drug discovery and developing a new medicine are a long, complex, costly and highly risky process with few peers in the commercial world. This is why computer-aided drug design (CADD) approaches are being widely used in the pharmaceutical industry to accelerate the process. The cost benefit of using computational tools in the lead optimization phase of drug development is substantial. On an average, it takes 10-15 years and millions of money to introduce a new drug into the market, with synthesis and testing of lead analogs being a large contributor to that sum [5]. Therefore, it is beneficial to apply computational tools in hit-to-lead optimization to cover a wider chemical space while reducing the number of compounds that must be synthesized and tested *in vitro*. The computational optimization of a hit compound involves a structure-based analysis of docking poses and energy profiles for hit analogs, ligand-based screening for compounds with similar chemical structure or improved predicted biological activity, or prediction of favorable affinity or optimize drug metabolism and pharmacokinetic properties such as absorption, distribution, metabolism, excretion and toxicity properties. The comparably low cost of CADD compared with chemical synthesis and biological characterization of compounds make these methods attractive to focus, reduce, and diversify the chemical space that is explored [6].

Bringing a new drug into the market is a costly process in terms of money, manpower, and time. Innovations in combinatorial chemistry that led to the increase of compound databases covering large chemical spaces aided in the expansion of drug discovery and the development of high-throughput screening (HTS) [2–3]. Despite this, the number of new molecular entities (NMEs) successfully launched into the market continued to decrease over the last several years [1]. To this end, employment of computer-aided drug discovery (CADD) techniques by top pharmaceutical companies and other research groups became crucial for the preliminary stage of drug discovery to dispatch the drug development process in a more cost-efficient way and to minimize failures in the final stage. Recent successes involving rational drug design have been reported elsewhere [4–6]. While HTS continues to be a big part of the drug discovery process in the pharmaceutical industry due to its high success rate, a lack of primary understanding of the molecular mechanism behind the activity of the identified hits can hamper the search of promising candidates [7–8].

The use of rational drug design, as applied in CADD, provides a knowledge-driven approach that can yield valuable information about the interaction pattern between protein and ligand (complex), as well as the binding affinity. In addition, the availability of supercomputers, parallel processing, and advanced software's have greatly promoted the rate of lead identification in pharmaceutical research.

The current scenario of the drug discovery process involves several disciplines such as chemical and structural biology, computational chemistry, organic synthesis, and pharmacology. Accordingly, it is comprised of several stages:

(a) **Target identification** involves the discovery and isolation of individual targets to investigate their functions and association with a specific disease [9].

(b) **Target validation** is the stage where the drug target is linked to the disease of interest, as well as their capacity to regulate biological functions in the body after binding to a partner molecule. Numerous studies are performed to ascertain that the target macromolecule is linked to the diseased state [10].

(c) **Lead identification** entails the discovery of a synthetic chemical that shows a degree of potency and specificity against a biological target and is assumed to have the makings of a drug that can cure the intended disease[11].

(d) **Lead optimization** covers the improvement of potency and other significant properties through iterative cycles of evaluation of the lead compound(s) and their analogs. Thus, both in vitro and in vivo experiments are conducted to prioritize and select candidates with optimum potential for development as a safe and efficient drug. Moreover, structure–activity relationships (SARs) are developed to determine pertinent pharmacokinetic and pharmacodynamics properties that can be applied to analogs that will be synthesized for evaluation [12].

(e) **Preclinical stage** involves drug synthesis and formulation research, in vivo animal studies for potency and toxicity, and characterization of mechanistic toxicity [13–14].

(f) **Clinical trials** include three phases that investigate the safety, adverse effects, dosage, efficacy, and pharmacokinetic properties of the candidate drug on human volunteers [14, 7].

Computational tools are useful for studying biological systems. There are a number of computational tools available to aid in the development of new pharmaceuticals. These computational tools may be useful during the rational development of novel pharmaceuticals and also for studying fundamental biological processes.

Ligand Based Drug Design

It is also known as indirect drug design. It relies on knowledge of other molecules that bind to the biological target of interest. These other molecules may be used to derive a pharmacophore model that defines the minimum necessary structural characteristics a molecule must possess in order to bind to the target [8]. Alternatively, a quantitative structure-activity relationship (QSAR), in which a correlation between the calculated properties of molecules and their experimentally determined biological activity, may be derived. These QSAR relationships in turn may be used to predict the activity of new analogs [9].

Structure Based Drug Design (SBDD)

It is known as direct drug design. Structure based drug design relies on structural knowledge of the target protein to design and optimize lead compounds. This knowledge is obtained from either experimental structures or computational predictions. A requirement is the availability of receptor structures:

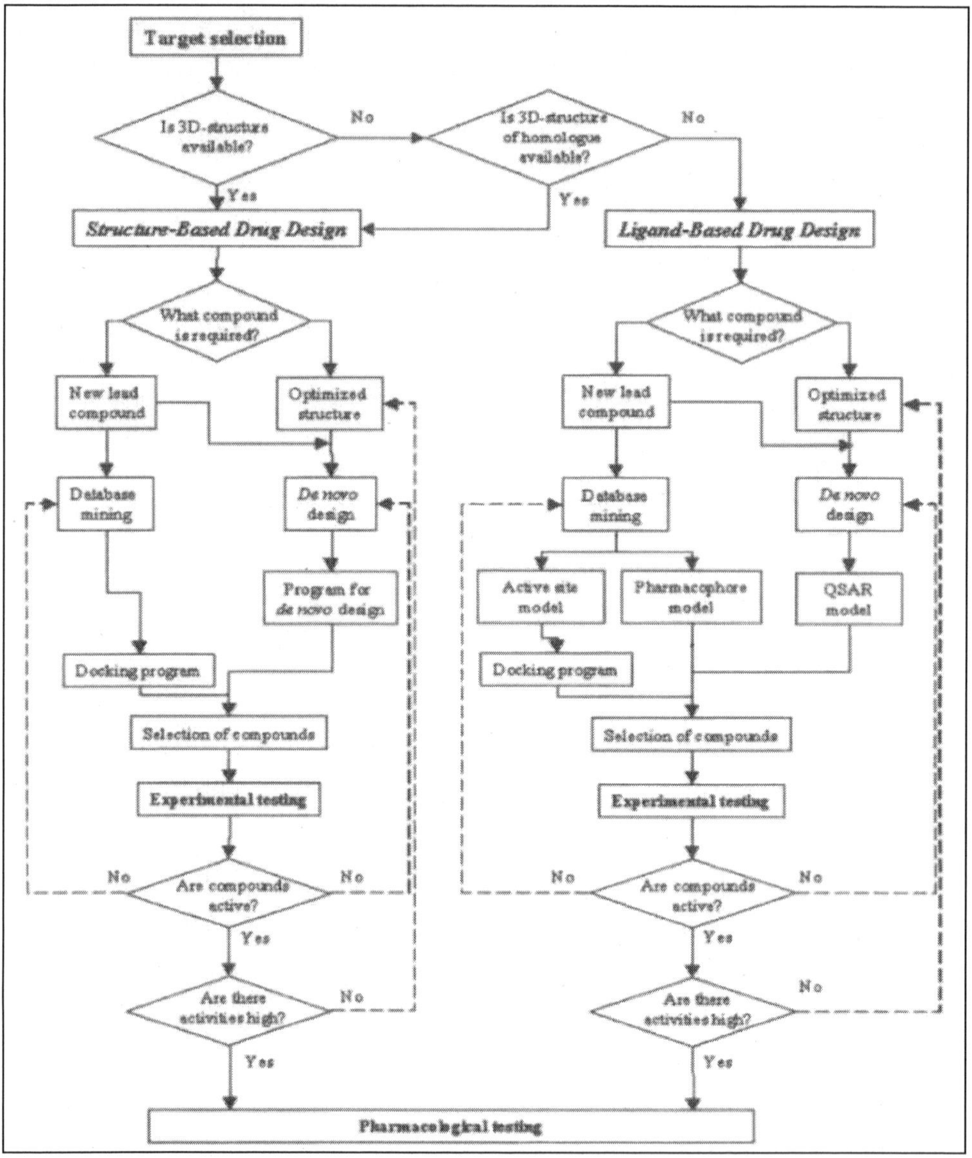

Figure 11.1: Overview of the Workflow of Computer Aided Drug Design [40].

1. NMR spectroscopy
2. X-ray crystallography

In practice protein X-ray crystallography is the major source of structural information. CADD can be separated into ligand or hit identification and ligand or hit optimization, with both structure based drug design and ligand based drug design methods useful in the appropriate context.

There are two basic strategies for searching of biologically active compounds by structure based drug design:

1. Molecular database mining for new ligands
2. Ligand design ***de novo***.

Molecular Database Mining

The modern superior approach in searching new lead structures implicates initial molecular database screening. The ground is the possibility for rather quicker selection and testing of numerous compounds. If compounds with desired activity have been discovered, they can be used for further modifications for piling up activity, decreasing side-effects and optimization of pharmacokinetic properties. The technique of searching in molecular databases is based upon the speculation that compounds with requested activity are synthesized earlier; even so they have been not tested for this particular activity. Thus, they can be found in databases. Several methods for molecular databases screening are applicable [37]. A remarkable method is the docking of compounds in active site of target. Various docking programs have been developed whereas DOCK is one of the widely used programs [38, 39]. Most algorithms of the docking programs use rigid structure of molecule-target. Usually preprocessing of a molecular database is carried out before the docking procedure. The compounds exhibiting patent properties (molecular mass, presence of the certain groups, similarity with known ligands, drug-likeness, *etc.*) are selected.

De Novo Drug Design

De novo means to start afresh, from the beginning, from the scratch. It is a process in which the 3D structure of receptor is used to design newer molecules. It involves the structural determination of the lead target complexes and lead modifications using molecular modeling tools. For the generation of drug molecules with desirable activity profiles towards a particular target biomolecule, structure based or ligand-based de novo design represents powerful approaches (**Figure 11.2**).

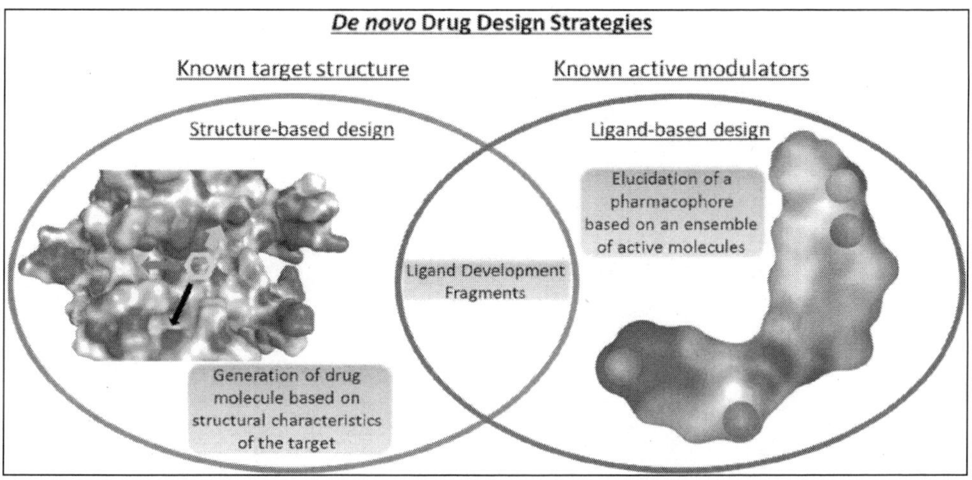

Figure 11.2: Design Strategies are Leading to Active and Selective Drug Molecules, Depending on the Knowledge available for the Biological Target [42].

Structure-Based De Novo Drug Design

With respect to the therapeutic target structure, a novel potential modulator can be designed into the binding site by placing single atoms at beneficial locations. In a force field, an initial atom, which is selected from a predefined set of atoms, gets randomly placed within the cavity as a seed from where the molecule grows by being connected to the next atom through a defined bond. As on every stage, a variety of atoms and different hybridization states of those atoms can be implemented, the chemical space covered by this approach is enormous and the output structures require being narrowed down by filtering according to parameters like chemical feasibility and structural uniqueness. The advantages of an atom by atom approach lie clearly in the huge chemical space that can be covered as well as in the high diversity of the generated structures. However, the weaknesses represented by the threat of combinatorial explosion of the output structures and the fact that many generated structures have to be discarded due to a lack of chemical accessibility need to be kept in mind when using this approach. Nishibata and Itai have developed LEGEND as a computational atom by atom de novo drug design tool [10].

To overcome the threats and shortcomings of an atom by atom approach, pre-defined fragments are used that preferentially lead to drafted molecules with high chemical feasibility. In this context, two approaches can be discerned for the design of novel structures:

a) Fragment-Linking
b) Fragment-Growing

a) Fragment-Linking

In this manner, by placing small fragments into the cavity, either computationally or by co-crystallization experiments, the pocket can be probed for constructive interactions between the fragment and the enzyme. In cases where the initial fragment derives from a screening campaign, it is necessary to be aware of the threat of false-positive hits [11]. The fragments are kept in the cavity and subsequently connected to each other via linker fragments as displayed in Figure 3. The connecting linker must have the correct length and geometry to bridge the distance between the fragments. Moreover, it has to fulfill the pharmacophore and the excluded volume defined in the initial query. Fragments and linkers are selected from databases that can be obtained either by virtual fragmentation of complete drug molecules or from external input such as catalogues of fragment-like compounds. The output structures are biased by the composition of the fragments and linkers in the database. The more diverse the collection is, the larger the covered chemical space gets.

b) Fragment Growing

In contrast, just one seed fragment is placed, computationally or by co-crystallization experiments, within the cavity of the biomolecule as a starting point following this method. By interacting with the active site, this seed is used as an anchor from which a novel ligand grows. Incorporation of small fragments during the growing process of the ligand leads to inhibitors displaying high diversity [13-21]. Compared to fragment-linking, the fragment-growing strategy provides more structural freedom at each stage as it is not limited to a repertoire of linkers to bridge the gap between two starting fragments with a given distance and angle in between [22].

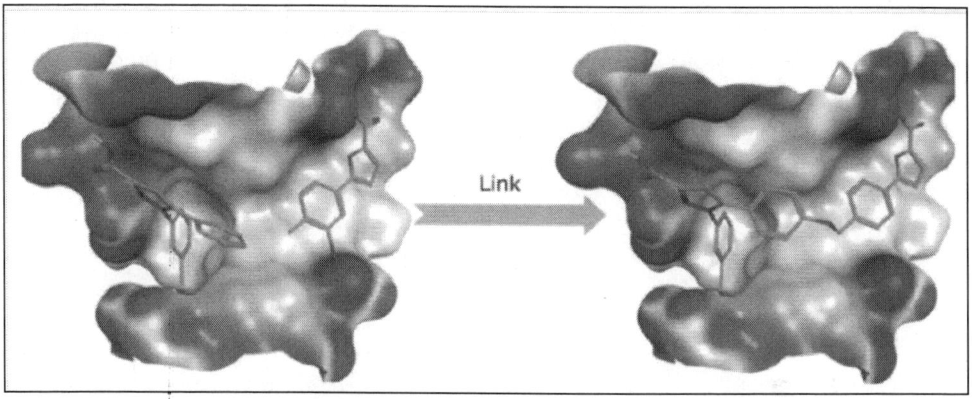

Figure 11.3: X-ray Structure of Two Individual Fragments in the Cavity of the N-terminal Domain of the 70 kDa Subunit of Replication Protein A (RPA70N), and a ligand that derived from linking the fragments. Ligand cartoons in green [12].

For computational fragment-based applications, LUDI, PROLIGAND, SPROUT, or CONCERTS are available software tools. If structural data of a ligand co-crystallized to its biological target is available, the scaffold of the ligand can be, erased leaving disconnected fragments in the pocket. In this case, the fragments can be re-connected by a linker, resulting in novel structures with a similar binding motif. This process of replacing a part of the molecule is known as scaffold replacement, scaffold hopping, or re-scaffolding [23-26].

Ligand-Based De Novo Drug Design

In the absence of the three-dimensional target structure, novel active compounds can still be designed when activity data for a set of known ligands are available [27]. These data usually come from screening campaigns or structure–activity relationship analyses and represent the basis of a ligand-based design approach. From an ensemble of active compounds, a common pharmacophore is defined and used to design novel compounds sharing the relevant features. A pitfall to be aware of is the possibility of diverse binding modes of different ligands. The main advantage of a ligand-based design approach lies in the fact that no crystallographic data needs to be in hand. This makes the method suitable for biological targets where crystallography is very challenging such as for the G protein-coupled receptors (GPCRs) [28]. Computational tools that allow ligand-based de novo drug design approaches include TOPAS, SYNOPSIS, and DOGS [29-30]. As enormous (virtual) databases are available, which include plenty of chemical structures and biological data, ligand-based virtual screening (LBVS) offers a path for mining this information and condense it to a subset of potentially active substances that are in consensus with pre-defined queries [31]. Such data mining for the identification of compounds with a certain set of descriptors is highly complex and requires sophisticated algorithms that are able to cope with big data. Over the past decades, artificial intelligence has evolved significantly and can be used to deal with massive amounts of data as found in drug discovery endeavors [32]. The techniques of machine learning and deep learning are used for both structure-based and ligand-based drug design [33,34]. Similarity searches, prediction of biological activity or ligand binding sites are possible with various machine learning techniques [35]. Nevertheless, as the selection of appropriate descriptors for computational processes as well as the evaluation of useful structures from a set of computer generated options still relies on the expertise of a human being, fully automated de novo drug design is still not on the horizon in the immediate future [36].

Active Site Modeling

Active site searching is an effective, computationally accessible method to identify compounds with qualities similar to that of an active, lead compound. For example, if the number of ligands for which biological activity is known are too few to build a QSAR model, active site searching may be effective. The most widely used descriptors in active site searching are chemical fingerprints or large numbers of physiochemical properties. To quantify the extent of similarity of active sites between compounds, different similarity measures are used alone or in combinations; these include the Tanimoto, Cosine, Hamming, Russel-Rao, and Forbes indices. Finally, it should be noted that it is useful to perform successive searches using the nearest neighbors of a query compound. A number of software packages, including MOE (Molecular Operating Environment, Chemical Computing Group) and Discovery Studio (Acclerys Inc) allow for similarity searching. Public small molecule databases such as PubChem ZINC and ChEMBL or open source software using those databases provide similarity searching and clustering tools.

Quantitative Structure-Activity Relationship (QSAR) Models

Quantitative structure-activity relationship (QSAR) models describe the mathematical relation between structural attributes and the target response of a set of chemicals [43]. Classic QSAR is known as the Hansch-Fujita approach and involves the correlation of various electronic, hydrophobic, and steric features with biologic activity. In the 1960s, Hansch (1964) and others began to establish QSAR models using various molecular descriptors to physical, chemical, and biologic properties focused on providing computational estimates for the bioactivity of molecules[44]. In 1964, Free and Wilson (1964) developed a mathematical model relating the presence of various chemical substituents to biologic activity (each type of chemical group was assigned an activity contribution), and the two methods were later combined to create the Hansch/Free-Wilson method. [45, 46]

The general workflow of a QSAR-based drug discovery project is to first collect a group of active and inactive ligands and then create a set of mathematical descriptors that describe the physicochemical and structural properties of those compounds. A model is then generated to identify the relationship between those descriptors and their experimental activity, maximizing the predictive power.

Finally, the model is applied to predict activity for a library of test compounds that were encoded with the same descriptors. Success of QSAR, therefore, depends not only on the quality of the initial set of active/inactive compounds but also on the choice of descriptors and the ability to generate the appropriate mathematical relationship. One of the most important considerations regarding this method is the fact that all models generated will be dependent on the sampling space of the initial set of compounds with known activity, the chemical diversity. In other words, divergent scaffolds or functional groups not represented within this "training" set of compounds will not be represented in the final model, and any potential hits within the library to be screened that contain these groups will likely be missed. Therefore, it is advantageous to cover a wide chemical space within the training set.

Pharmacophore Modelling

Pharmacophore approaches are successful subfields of computer-aided drug design (CADD) which have become one of the major tools in hit identification, lead optimization, and rational design of novel drugs [41]. In 1998, the International Union of Pure and Applied Chemistry (IUPAC) formally defined a pharmacophore as "the ensemble of steric and electronic features that is necessary to ensure the optimal supra-molecular interactions with a specific biological target structure and to trigger (or to block) its biological response". A pharmacophore model explains how structurally diverse ligands can bind to a common receptor site [41]. Furthermore, pharmacophore models can be used to identify through de novo design or virtual screening novel ligands that will bind to the same receptor [41].

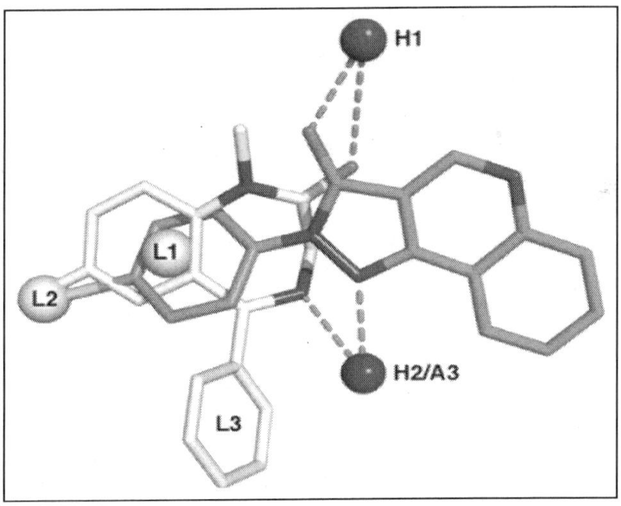

Figure 11.4: An Example of a Pharmacophore Model of the Benzodiazepine Binding Site on the GABA Receptor [41].

White sticks represent the carbon atoms of the benzodiazepine diazepam, while green represents carbon atoms of the non benzodiazepine CGS-9896. Red and blue sticks are oxygen and nitrogen atoms that are present in both structures [41]. The red spheres labeled H1 and H2/A3 are, respectively, hydrogen bond donating and accepting sites in the receptor, while L1, L2, and L3 denote lipophilic binding sites [41].

The process for developing a pharmacophore model principally involves the following steps:

1. **Select a Training Set of Ligands:** A structurally diverse set of molecules is chosen that will be used for developing the pharmacophore model. As a pharmacophore model should be able to discriminate between molecules with and without bioactivity, the set of molecules should include both active and inactive compounds.
2. **Conformational Analysis:** A set of low energy conformations is generated that is likely to contain the bioactive conformation for each of the selected molecules.
3. **Molecular Superimposition:** All combinations of the low-energy conformations of the molecules are superimposed. Similar (bioisosteric) functional groups common to all molecules in the set might be fitted (For example, phenyl rings or carboxylic acid groups). The set of conformations (one conformation from each active molecule) that results in the best fit is presumed to be the active conformation.
4. **Abstraction:** The superimposed molecules are transferred into an abstract representation. For example, superimposed phenyl rings might be referred to more conceptually as an 'aromatic ring' pharmacophore element. Correspondingly, hydroxy groups could be designated as a 'hydrogen-bond donor/acceptor' pharmacophore element.
5. **Validation:** A pharmacophore model is a *hypothesis* accounting for the observed biological activities of a set of molecules that bind to a common biological target. The model is only valid insofar as it is able to account for differences in the biological activity of a range of molecules.

When the biological activities of new molecules become available, the pharmacophore model can be updated to further refine it. [41]

Conclusion

The computer-aided drug design portrays a sophisticated discipline using achievement in various fields of science and various methods and approaches. The perpetuity of strategies in drug discovery ranges from serendipity. It has repeatedly provided amazing insights during rational drug discovery projects, to machine-based learning, which is the other extreme of the strategies. Undoubtedly CADD needs several basic data: 3D structure of target, or its homologues, and also sets of ligands. If such information is not available the only way is experimental methods. The high-throughput screening is optimal method for discovery of active compounds for new targets. However, structure-based docking is preferred over random screening only when the 3D structure of target is recognized. In a nutshell, the methods and approaches associated in CADD look simple, absolute and comprehensive [47].

REFERENCES

1. Augen, J. Drug Discov. Today, 2002, 7, 315.
2. Lohse, M.J. Trends Pharmacol. Sci., 1998, 19, 198.
3. Borchardt, J.K. The Alchemist 6 December 2001,http: //www.chemweb.com/alchem/articles/10059288538
4. A.V. Veselovsky* and A.S. Ivanov; V. N. Orekhovich Institute of Biomedical Chemistry, Russian Academy of Medical Science, 2003, Pogodinskaya str., 10, Moscow, 119121, Russia, 33.
5. Basak SC. Chemobioinformatics: the advancing frontier of computer-aided drug design in the post-genomic era. Curr. Comput. Aided. Drug. Des. 2012;8: 1-2.
6. Enyedy IJ and Egan WJ. Can we use docking and scoring for hit-to-lead optimization? J. Comput. Aided. Mol. Des. 2008;22: 161-168.n
7. Role of computer-aided drug design in modern drug discovery; Stephani, Joy Y. Macalino, Vijayakumar Gosu, Sunhye Hong, Sun Choi;(DOI 10.1007/s12272-015-0640-5)
8. *Guner OF (2000). Pharmacophore Perception, Development, and use in Drug Design. La Jolla, Calif: International University Line.* ISBN 978-0-9636817-6-8.
9. *Tropsha A (2010).* "QSAR in Drug Discovery". *In Reynolds CH, Merz KM, Ringe D (eds.). Drug Design: Structure- and Ligand-Based Approaches (1 ed.). Cambridge, UK: Cambridge University Press. pp. 151–164.* ISBN 978-0521887236.
10. Nishibata Y, Itai A. Automatic creation of drug candidate structures based on receptor structure. Starting point for artificial lead generation. Tetrahedron 1991;47: 8985–8990.
11. Cramer J, Schiebel J, Wulsdorf T, *et al.*, A false-positive screening hit in fragment-based lead discovery: watch out for the red herring. Angew. Chem. Int. Ed. 2017;56: 1908–1913; Angew. Chem. 2017;129: 1934–1940.
12. Frank AO, Feldkamp MD, Kennedy JP, *et al.*, Discovery of a potent inhibitor of replication protein a protein–protein interactions using a fragment-linking approach. J. Med. Chem. 2013;56: 9242–9250.
13. Ichihara O, Barker J, Law RJ, *et al.*, Compound design by fragment-linking. Mol. Inform. 2011;30: 298–306.
14. Schneider G. Future de novo drug design. Mol. Inform. 2014;33: 397–402.
15. Schneider P, Schneider G. De novo design at the edge of chaos. J. Med. Chem. 2016;59: 4077–4086.
16. Hartenfeller M, Schneider G. Enabling future drug discovery by de novo design. Wiley Interdiscip. Rev. Comput. Mol. Sci. 2011;1: 742–759.
17. Lanz J, Riedl R. Merging allosteric and active site binding motifs: de novo generation of target selectivity and potency via natural-product-derived fragments. ChemMedChem 2015;10: 451–454.

18. Chevillard F, Rimmer H, Betti C, *et al.,* Binding-site compatible fragment growing applied to the design of β2-adrenergic receptor ligands. J. Med. Chem. 2018;61: 1118–1129.

19. Liu T, Naderi M, Alvin C, *et al.,* Break down in order to build up: decomposing small molecules for fragment-based drug design with eMolFrag. J. Chem. Inf. Model. 2017;57: 627–631.

20. Esposito C, Wiedmer L, Caflisch A. In silico identification of JMJD3 demethylase inhibitors. J. Chem. Inf. Model. 2018;58: 2151–2163.

21. Dey F, Caflisch A. Fragment-based de novo ligand design by multiobjective evolutionary optimization. J. Chem. Inf. Model. 2008;48: 679–690.

22. Hung AW, Silvestre HL, Wen S, *et al.,* Application of fragment growing and fragment linking to the discovery of inhibitors of Mycobacterium tuberculosis pantothenate synthetase. Angew. Chem. Int. Ed. 2009;48: 8452–8456; Angew. Chem. 2009;121: 8604–8608

23. Böhm H-J, Flohr A, Stahl M. Scaffold hopping. Drug Discov. Today Technol. 2004;1: 217–224.

24. Schneider G, Schneider P, Renner S. Scaffold-hopping: how far can you jump? QSAR Comb. Sci. 2006;25: 1162–1171.

25. Sun H, Tawa G, Wallqvist A. Classification of scaffold hopping approaches. Drug Discov. Today 2012;17: 310–324.

26. Langdon SR, Ertl P, Brown N. Bioisosteric replacement and scaffold hopping in lead generation and optimization. Mol. Inform. 2010;29: 366–385.

27. Wang Y, Zhao H, Brewer JT, *et al.,* De novo design, synthesis, and biological evaluation of 3,4-disubstituted pyrrolidine sulfonamides as potent and selective glycine transporter 1 competitive inhibitors. J. Med. Chem. 2018;61: 7486–7502.

28. Levit A, Barak D, Behrens M, *et al.,* Homology model-assisted elucidation of binding sites in GPCRs. In: editors, Vaidehi N, KleinSeetharaman J. Membrane protein structure and dynamics. Methods in molecular biology (methods and protocols). Vol. 914. Totowa, NJ: Humana Press; 2012;179–205.

29. Hartenfeller M, Zettl H, Walter M, *et al.,* DOGS: reaction-driven de novo design of bioactive compounds. PLoS Comput. Biol. 2012;8: e1002380.

30. Schneider G, Lee M-L, Stahl M, *et al.,* De novo design of molecular architectures by evolutionary assembly of drug-derived building blocks. J. Comput. Aided Mol. Des. 2000;14: 487–494

31. Vinkers HM, de Jonge MR, Daeyaert FFD, *et al.,* SYNOPSIS: synthesize and optimize system in silico. J. Med. Chem. 2003;46: 2765–2773.

32. Lavecchia A. Machine-learning approaches in drug discovery: methods and applications. Drug Discov. Today 2015;20: 318–331.

33. Zhang L, Tan J, Han D, *et al.,* From machine learning to deep learning: progress in machine intelligence for rational drug discovery. Drug Discov. Today 2017;22: 1680–1685.

34. Gawehn E, Hiss JA, Schneider G. Deep learning in drug discovery. Mol. Inform. 2016;35: 3–14

35. Lima AN, Philot EA, Trossini GHG, *et al.*, Use of machine learning approaches for novel drug discovery. Expert Opin. Drug Discov. 2016;11: 225–239.

36. Schneider G, Clark DE. Automated de novo drug design – "Are we nearly there yet?". Angew. Chem. Int. Ed. 2019. Accepted Author Manuscript. DOI: 10.1002/anie.201814681.

37. Weber, H.P. In Computer-Aided Drug Design Industrial Research, Herrmann, E.C.; Franke, R. Eds. Springer Verlag: Berlin. 1995, pp. 111-128.

38. Kuntz, I.D.; Blaney, J.M.; Oatley, S.J.; Landridge, R.; Ferrin, T.E. J. Mol. Biol., 1982, 161, 269.

39. Ewing T.J.A.; Makino S.; Skillman A.G.; Kuntz, I.D. J. Comp.-Aided Mol. Design, 2001, 15, 411.

40. A.V. Veselovsky and A.S. Ivanov; Current Drug targets. Infectious Disorders, 01 Mar 2003, 3(1): 33; DOI: 10.2174/1568005033342145, PMID: 12570731.

41. https: //www.profacgen.com/pharmacophore-modeling.htm

42. Thomas Fischer, Silvia Gazzola and Rainer Riedl (2019) Approaching Target Selectivity by De Novo Drug Design, Expert Opinion on Drug Discovery, 14: 8, 792, DOI: 10.1080/17460441.2019.1615435.

43. Zhang S Methods Mol Biol. 2011; 716: (23-38). Computer-aided drug discovery and development.

44. Hansch C. (1964), J Amer Chem Soc 86: (1616–1626). Rho-Sigma-Pi-analysis—a method for the correlation of biological-activity and chemical-structure.

45. FREE SM Jr, WILSON JW. J Med Chem. 1964 Jul; 7: (395-9). A MATHEMATICAL CONTRIBUTION TO STRUCTURE-ACTIVITY STUDIES.

46. Tmej C, Chiba P, Huber M, Richter E, Hitzler M, Schaper KJ, Ecker G.Arch Pharm (Weinheim). 1998 Jul-Aug; 331(7-8): 233-40. A combined Hansch/ Free-Wilson approach as predictive tool in QSAR studies on propafenone-type modulators of multidrug resistance.

47. Wolber G, Seidel T, Bendix F, Langer T. Drug Discov Today. 2008 Jan; 13(1-2): 23-9. Molecule-pharmacophore superpositioning and pattern matching in computational drug design.

Chapter 12

Methods of Euthanasia

The word **euthanasia** means an easy death and should be regarded as an act of humane killing with the minimum of pain, fear, and distress.

Biomedical research needs animals in case of in-vivo animal experiments. For other scientific purposes *e.g., in vitro* studies, the biological material is also necessary to study enzymes, membranes, receptors, cells, tissues, or organs which are obtained from dead animals.

Euthanasia procedures must be performed by persons competent in and qualified for the methods to be used or under the direct supervision of a competent person. Some methods require considerable training and experience to be used appropriately.

Training should include:

- Familiarity with the normal behaviour of the species being euthanased
- An appreciation of how handling and restraint affect behaviour
- An understanding of the mechanisms by which the selected technique induces loss of consciousness and death
- Recognition of signs of pain and distress.

The following criteria should be necessary for euthanasia:

- Is painless
- Produces rapid loss of consciousness and death
- Interrupts consciousness and reflexes simultaneously
- Requires minimum restraint
- Avoids excitement and causes minimal psychological stress to the animals
- Is appropriate for the age of the animal
- Exhibits consistent and predictable action

- ☆ Is easily and safely administered by properly trained personnel
- ☆ Causes minimal emotional effects to operator and observers
- ☆ Is not a disease or environmental problem
- ☆ It does not result in tissue changes that would affect a post-mortem diagnosis
- ☆ Is economical and readily available
- ☆ It does not leave carcasses

Techniques of Euthansia

Chemical Method
- Inhalant
- Injectables

Physical Method
- Shooting
- Penetrating Captive-Bolt Pistols
- Decapitation
- Cervical dislocation
- Stunning
- Exsanguination
- Pithing
- Microwave Irradiation

I. Physical Methods

1. Shooting

Shooting is a quick and effective means of humanely destroying animals and in most situations is the only practical method available for use in the field. Head shots are preferred when euthanasing animals that are immobilised by injury or physical restraint. Correctly placed head shots cause brain function to cease and result in an instantaneous loss of consciousness. Shooting should only be performed by skilled operators who have the necessary experience with firearms and who hold the appropriate licences and accreditation. Rifles, handguns and shotguns are used for this purpose [1].

2. Penetrating Captive-Bolt Pistols

A penetrating captive-bolt pistol uses a blank cartridge to fire a bolt into the brain of the animal. This causes concussion and trauma to the cerebral hemispheres and brainstem, which renders the animal instantaneously unconscious. In some cases the animal may not die quickly, therefore, it is recommended that immediately after the procedure, death of the animal is ensured by a second procedure such as exsanguination or pithing. It is an acceptable method of euthanasia in larger animals ie horses, pigs and ruminants (sheep, cattle, goats *etc.*).The procedure must be followed by a properly trained operator [2].

3. Stunning by a Blow to the Gead

Stunning the animal by a blow to the head may be acceptable in small or young animals with a soft skull (*e.g.* neonatal pigs, rats, mice, kittens, newborn pups, birds, reptiles, amphibians, fish). A single, sharp blow should be delivered to the central skull bones. This can be achieved with a hard and heavy, blunt instrument (*e.g.* metal pipe, wooden club *etc.*). Stunning must be immediately followed by a second method that ensures death (*e.g.* exsanguination, cervical dislocation, pithing). If not performed correctly, various degrees of consciousness with accompanying pain can occur [3].

4. Cervical Dislocation

This method involves the separation of the skull and the brain from the spinal cord by pressure applied posterior to the base of the skull. The brain stem which controls respiration and heart activity is consequently damaged, stopping breathing and reducing blood flow to the brain, leading to death. This method is used in small animals such as rodents and rabbits. A skilled operator is required to perform this technique [4].

5. Decapitation

Decapitation involves the rapid severing of the head from the body using a guillotine or sharp blade. Violent muscular contraction can occur after decapitation. This method is an acceptable method for very small mammals. [5]

6 Exsanguination

Exsanguination or 'bleeding out' of the carcass is achieved by cutting the major blood vessels in the neck (ie the carotid arteries and jugular veins). Exsanguination must not be used as a sole method of euthanasia as extreme hypovolemia is associated with anxiety. This method is not acceptable for birds because of the tendency for the blood to clot relatively quickly and thus result in incomplete bleeding-out. It is also not acceptable for reptiles and other cold-blooded vertebrates because of their slow metabolic rate and tolerance to hypoxia. It should only be used on unconscious animals *i.e.* those that have been stunned or anesthetized [6].

7. Pithing

Pithing is sometimes used as an adjunctive procedure to ensure death in an animal that has been rendered unconscious by other means (*e.g.* stunning). It is carried out by inserting a sharp needle or probe through the foramen magnum into the base of the brain to ensure brain destruction. Pithing can also be performed by inserting a probe through the hole made by a captive bolt. This method is used for some fish, amphibians and reptiles.

8. Microwave Irradiation

Euthanasia by microwave irradiation is used by neurobiologists for fixation of brain metabolites without destruction of brain anatomy. Specific equipment must be used for this purpose. It is essential to localize correctly the microwave beam onto the brain of the animal.

II. Chemical Methods

1. Inhalant Agents

Euthanasia with inhaled gases is slow due to the requirement for any gas being inhaled to reach the required concentration in the tissues before taking effect. A closed chamber for holding the gas is needed and personnel safety must be considered in order to avoid exposure to the toxic gas.

Carbon dioxide (CO_2): Carbon dioxide used in a sealed environment is suitable for animals up to 3 kg and is mostly used for small birds and rodents.When animals are placed into a chamber containing up to 70 per cent CO_2 they lose consciousness very quickly due to the narcotic effect of the high intake of CO_2 on the brain without causing hypoxia. Death is caused by direct depression of CNS, respiratory and cardiac functions.

Carbon monoxide (CO): When inhaled, carbon monoxide binds to haemoglobin in the red blood cells, with an affinity 250 times that of oxygen. This results in reduced oxygen-carrying capacity and altered delivery of oxygen to cells. Hypoxia - the reduction of oxygen supply to the tissues - eventually leads to unconsciousness and death. Death occurs rapidly at CO concentrations of 4 to 6 per cent. Carbon monoxide concentrations greater than 2 per cent are sufficient to cause loss of consciousness within minutes. Failure of the respiratory center then occurs followed by death from cardiac arrest.

Anesthetic gases: Halothane and the halogenated ethers, for example, isoflurane, methoxyflurane can be used with small animals (< 7kg). The animal can be placed in a sealed chamber containing cotton or gauze soaked with an appropriate amount of an anesthetic or the anesthetic vapour can be introduced from a vaporizer into the container or a plastic bag that has been placed around a cage containing the animal. The animal will become unconscious quickly.

2 Injectable Agents

Barbiturates: One of the most suitable methods of euthanasia is the administration of a barbiturate overdose either by the intravenous, intraperitoneal or intra cardiac routes. Injections by the intraperitoneal route work much more slowly than the intravenous route but are easier for an operator working alone. The intraperitoneal route is used when an intravenous injection would result in stressful handling or be dangerous to the animal or the operator and when there are no easily accessible veins. Intra cardiac injection should only be used if the animal is heavily sedated, unconscious or anesthetized.

Ideal Euthanizing Agent

- Not cause anxiety, fear, vocalization muscular spasm
- Painless
- Fast acting
- Reliable (work properly every time)
- Safe and easy to use for the properly trained person

- Economical
- Not pollute environment
- Practical to use

Signs of Death

- After the application of a euthanasia procedure, it is essential that the death of the animal be confirmed.
- Absence of respiratory movement.
- Absence of heart beat.
- Absence of pulse.
- Loss of colour in mucous membranes.
- Corneal and palpebral reflexes are lost.
- Glazing of eyes.

Disposal of Carcasses

Carcasses should only be discarded once death has been established. Carcasses should be disposed of properly and in accordance with acceptable practices. If the carcass presents a risk to wildlife (*e.g.* it contains infectious disease agents or residues of euthanasia chemicals) it should be disposed of by incineration or by burying in a deep hole after covering with lime. If large numbers of animals are to be killed, provisions should be made to dispose of carcasses in an appropriate manner.

Table 12.1: Recommended Methods of Euthanasia for a Range of Species

Sl.No.	*Species*	*Physical Methods*	*Chemical Methods*
1.	Amphibians	Stunning followed by decapitation	Gassing with carbon dioxide for >4 hours Overdose of barbiturate
2.	Bats and flying foxes		Inhalation of anesthetic gases or CO_2 Overdose of barbiturate
3.	Birds (large size) *e.g.* emu, ibis	Shooting	Overdose of barbiturate
4.	Birds (small to medium size) *e.g.* starlings, mynas, cockatoos, galahs	Neck (cervical) dislocation. Shooting (with shotgun)	Inhalation of anesthetic gases or CO_2 Overdose of barbiturate
5.	Cats	Shooting	Inhalation of anesthetic gases or CO_2 Overdose of barbiturate
6.	Cattle/Buffalo	Shooting Captive bolt stunning	Overdose of barbiturate
7.	Crocodiles	Shooting	Overdose of barbiturate
8.	Deer	Shooting	Overdose of barbiturate
9.	Dogs	Shooting	Overdose of barbiturate

Sl.No.	Species	Physical Methods	Chemical Methods
10.	Goats	Shooting Captive bolt stunning	Overdose of barbiturate
11.	Horses/Donkeys	Shooting Captive bolt stunning	Overdose of barbiturate
12.	Pigs	Shooting Captive bolt stunning Stunning by a blow to the head followed by exsanguination	Overdose of barbiturate
13.	Rabbits/Hares	Cervical dislocation Shooting	Overdose of barbiturate Inhalation of anesthetic gases or CO_2
14.	Rodents	Cervical dislocationStunning plus exsanguination	Inhalation of anesthetic gases or CO_2 Overdose of barbiturate
15.	Reptiles - snakes and lizards	Stunning/decapitation/destruction of the brain Shooting	
16.	Reptiles - tortoises and turtles	Stunning/decapitation/destruction of the brain Shooting	Overdose of barbiturate
17.	Sheep	Shooting Captive bolt stunning Exsanguination (or bleeding out)	Overdose of barbiturate

REFERENCES

1. Trudy Sharp. Methods of euthanasia. https: //www.cabi.org/isc.
2. Neville Gregory and Frank Shaw. Penetrating Captive Bolt Stunning and Exsanguination of Cattle in Abattoirs. 04 Jun 2010 Pages 215-230. https: //doi.org/10.1207/S15327604JAWS0303_3.
3. John E. Cooper, Anesthesia, Analgesia, and Euthanasia of Invertebrates, *ILAR Journal*, Volume 52, Issue 2, 2011, Pages 196–204, https: //doi.org/10.1093/ilar.52.2.196.
4. Terson de Paleville, Daniela G L *et al.*, "Respiratory motor control disrupted by spinal cord injury: mechanisms, evaluation, and restoration." *Translational stroke research* vol. 2,4 (2011): 463-73. doi: 10.1007/s12975-011-0114-0
5. Jiménez-Coello, Matilde *et al.*, 'Medical and Bioethical Issues in Laboratory Animal.' Euthanasia: The 'Good Death' Controversy in Humans and Animals, edited by Josef Kuøe, InTech, 2011, pp. 191-218.
6. Karl J.Campbel.The next generation of rodent eradications: Innovative technologies and tools to improve species specificity and increase their feasibility on islands. Biological Conservation.Vol 185, May 2015, pp. 47-58.

Appendix I

Hematological Values of Laboratory Animals

	Mouse	*Rat*	*Hamster*	*G. Pig*	*Rabbit*	*Cat*	*Dog (Beagle)*	*Monkey (Rhesus)*
RBC ($\times 10^6/mm^3$)	7-12.5	7-10	6-10	4.5-7	4-7	5-10	5.5-8.5	3.5-6.9
PCV (per cent)	39-49	36-18	36-55	37-48	36-48	30-15	37-55	26-48
Hb (g/dL)	10.2-16.6	11-18	10-16	11-15	10-15.5	8-15	12-18	8.8-16.5
WBC ($\times 10^3/mm^3$)	6-15	6-17	3-11	7-18	9-11	5.5-19.5	6-17	2.5-26.7
Neutrophils (per cent)	10-40	9-34	10-42	28-44	20-75	35-75	60-70	5-88
Lymphocytes (per cent)	55-95	65-85	50-95	39-72	30-85	20-55	12-30	8-92
Eosinophils (per cent)	0-4	0-6	0-4.5	1-5	0-4	2-12	2-10	0-14
Monocytes (per cent)	0.1-35	0-5	0-3	3-12	1-4	1-4	3-10	0-11
Basophils (per cent)	0-0.3	0-1.5	0-1	0-3	2-7	Rare	rare	0-6
Platelets ($\times 10^3/mm^3$)	160-410	500-1300	200-500	250-850	250-656	300-700	200-900	109-597

RBC = red blood cells, PCV = packed cell volume, WBC = white blood cells, Hb = hemoglobin

Note: The range of normal values may vary in a laboratory using specific species, strain, and sub strain of these animals.

Source: CPCSEA guide line for laboratory animal facility.

Biochemical Values of Laboratory Animals

	Mouse	*Rat*	*Hamster*	*G. Pig*	*Rabbit*	*Cat*	*Dog*	*Monkey*
Total protein (g/dl)	3.5-7.2	5.6-7.6	4.5-7.5	4.6-6.2	5.4-7.5	6-7.5	6-7.5	4.9-9.3
Albumin (g/dl)	2.5-4.8	2.8-4.8	2.6-4.1	2.1-3.9	2.7-4.6	2.5-4.0	3-4	2.8-5.2
Globulin (g/dl)	0.6	1.8-3	2.7-4.2	1.7-2.6	1.5-2.8	2.5-3.8	2.4-3.7	1.2-5.8
Glucose (mg/dl)	62-175	50-135	60-150	60-125	75-150	81-108	54-99	46-178
BUN (mg/dl)	12-28	15-21	12-25	9-31.5	17-23.5	3.5-8.0	3.5-7.5	8-40
Creatinine (mg/dl)	0.3-1	0.2-0.8	0.91-0.99	0.6-2.2	0.8-1.8	180	120 (nmol/l)	0.1-2.8 (nmol/l)
Bilirubin (mg/dl)	0.1-0.9	0.2-0.55	0.25-0.6	0.3-0.9	0.25-0.74	4.0	5.0 (mmol/l)	0.1-2 (nmol/l)
Cholesterol (mg/dl)	26-82	40-130	25-135	20-43	35-53	2-4	4-7 (mmol/l)	108-263 (mmol/l)

Note: The range of normal values may vary in a laboratory using specific species, strain, and sub strain of these animals.

Source: CPCSEA guide line for laboratory animal facility.

Index